FOREWORDS

D0324888

Johanna is a refreshing expert in the area of wellbeing. Simply stated, she is a guru of how to live vibrantly, how to shed weight, increase energy and improve the natural flow of life that pulses through the body. "Live Vibrantly! 10 Steps To Maintain Youthfulness, Increase Energy, Restore Your Health" is a guide for anyone willing to adjust their thinking to a paradigm of wellness and away from the collective consciousness focused on dis-ease (disease is merely a state of being without ease).

According to the World Health Organization, the worldwide pharmaceutical industry is a $300 billion a year market...and growing. Every ailment or potential dis-ease has a pill and none of it is in harmony with the natural energy of the body. Vibrancy, life, energy and wellbeing do not come from pills. Johanna shows you how to live every day with energy, avoid illness and increase your state of being well through the foods you choose. Johanna guides you to an understanding of health sourced from nature and the alignment of all nature to living vibrantly.

What we eat either gives us life or depletes us. Johanna guides us to live vibrantly through the food choices we make. She is passionate about helping each person she works with create a new level of energy and health.

My fiancée and I brought Johanna into our home for a week to teach us about preparing foods which promote health and energy. During her time with us we learned how to select and prepare foods that increased the level of natural energy we felt. Johanna doesn't force feed you into adopting a "good for you" approach with foods that are hard to swallow. Let's face it, if something is good for you but is not pleasant to eat, most people will give up on what is best for them and opt for the immediate gratification of the food-like substitutes most people eat these days. Johanna's approach is to teach you how to choose, prepare and enjoy foods that will give you life!

I live vibrantly thanks to Johanna's knowledge and passionate commitment to showing others how to achieve wellness, energy and vibrancy.

Mark Dannenberg: Entrepreneur, Author, Options Trader, Host of the Elite Trader Live Trading Room

Live Vibrantly! 10 Steps To Maintain Youthfulness, Increase Energy, Restore Your Health

It's always a special moment when someone asks me to write a Foreword, to be given an opportunity to present someone's mission to the world. More specifically, it's momentous IF the book's material is particularly insightful, innovative, cutting edge, worthwhile, caring, truly informative and well done. Yes, that's a special moment because suddenly the invited Foreword writer becomes a de facto genius, illuminated by the author's brilliance. But most specifically of all, it's a special moment when, after reading the book, there's a certain gut feeling, a feeling in one's marrow, that affirms, "this message is worthy of widespread dissemination into the human collective consciousness, and I'm compelled to help share this blessing."

This is that most special moment.

So to provide you with a proper Fore-word or two, let me first attest to the author's dedication and competency, and then Fore-tell what you will soon discern as apparent—"Live Vibrantly! 10 Steps To Maintain Youthfulness, Increase Energy, Restore Your Health" will inspire you to find great joy in the simple, profound steps that will help you live in the most optimal health possible. It's a genuine survival guide for the 21st Century.

In the 21st Century, we find that humanity is becoming absorbed with minutiae. If a health pundit says, "Eat sweet potatoes, they're good for you," people will ask, "Can I eat it before noon in the moon's gibbous phase; how many times must I chew it to activate amylase; is it better to steam it and not bake; can I put 15 chia seeds on it if the seeds are raw; does it have enough resistant starch to support my microbiota but not cause a SIBO/FODMAPS/GERD/GAPS/CELIAC cross-reactive histamine/oxalate reaction; and can I combine it with green beans even though the colors might clash?

There's a reason for the excessive, fastidious attention on minutiae. It's born of suffering—born of seeking solutions for the damage of refined, processed foods; the constant poisoning that antibiotics in commercial meat and dairy products cause to our allies in health, the gut microbiota; for the aberrant insults that genetically modified and glyphosate pesticides in food cause to the intestinal lining that breaks the natural order from our cells.

Humanity can't win a conflict of minutiae where health factors become more numerous than the stars, but we can go back to ten simple Steps To Maintain Youthfulness, Increase Energy, Restore Your Health. That's what this book is about—simple, commonsense, profound steps that define a healthy lifestyle. If we embrace that which is good for us, we don't have to worry so much about all the things that are bad … we'll just keep them away from our sacrosanct temples, and prosper by being in accord with Nature.

The destiny of humanity is to move onward and upward in the realms of heart, mind and spirit, but we cannot neglect the body because it's part of the whole. After the great strides of the Renaissance and Age of Enlightenment, the perversions that line the grocery store shelves are forcing humanity back to the "bovine" mentality of having to spend 90% of our time grazing on minutiae, worrying, and seeking solutions for food toxins and the body's reactions to altered foods. Unnatural practices have not only "dumbed down" our mental vibrancy, for example, with fluoride in the water supply, they've forced the disease label, *orthorexia nervosa*, on people who simply wish to be healthy and understand that "their bodies are what they eat."

In this book, Johanna provides simple solutions so we can get our noses out of the manure and once again look to the heavens and embrace the sublime. Once you engage its tenets, you won't have to 'sweat the small stuff.' Now that's powerful!

There is a profound simplicity to Nature and thus also a profound simplicity to the body's basic needs for food, water, sunshine, air, sleep, and nurture. Would you like to set up a lifeline, e.g. your kitchen, to connect you to Nature's bounty, relax, and enjoy having a wide variety of foods without all the worry about the ever-shifting opinions bantered about by health pundits? Is it not better to trust Natural Law than to trust fads and trends? Johanna's steps are founded on Natural Law and that law says that you can once again eat spaghetti and slather dressing all over your salad. She's figured out how to dodge the myriad tar traps of modern life and keep your feet on the safe path. Here's your golden ticket to freedom.

Johanna is a person who lives and breathes the natural health ideals, and most importantly she puts them into practice. But best of all, she "gets it." She first pays homage to the Natural Laws that govern life and health, and then applies Nature's "Law of Economy" that puts the most nutrition for the least amount of effort right on the plate.

If you take her 10 Steps and integrate each one into your daily life, and make them your "status quo," you'll have a strong foundation upon which to build your health and experience the rewards that a vibrant body, mind, and spirit bring. She'll show you how.

We all seek that peaceful, calm, joyous contentment in a world of cacophonous jangles. Knowing how to support our health with grace and ease is foundational to being who we really are. This book moves beyond the confusions and provides a way to take charge of your health, your cells and microbiome, so you can indeed "live health" and get on with fulfilling your purpose in life with energy and acuity.

It's with great gratitude that I've been allowed to present the virtues of Johanna's information as an appetizer for what's to come. Best wishes in your natural health endeavors!

WellnessWiz Jack Tips (Ph.D., C.C.N.)

Live Vibrantly! 10 Steps To Maintain Youthfulness, Increase Energy, Restore Your Health

TESTIMONIALS

"Johanna helped me adjust my diet and opened my eyes to the benefits of good nutrition when I was struggling with arthritis. I explained my issues to Johanna, she listened well, and with the guidance she gave I made significant changes to the way that I eat. Then over a period of 6 months I actually managed to push my arthritis into remission on nutritional changes alone. Johanna is a great nutritionist and this is a very easy recommendation to make..."

John Fry

Johanna provided me with the deepest dive personal nutrition plan I have ever had. She coupled her intricate knowledge of how nutrition impacts personal systems biology with my current eating habits and lifestyle to come up with a highly actionable and achievable set of recommendations. I would particularly recommend Johanna if you are already highly conscious of your health and wellness, and want someone to help you optimize.

Zak Holdsworth

"Johanna has created an innovative and insightful program, called 'Breeze Through Menopause,' applying advanced nutritional concepts and traditional foods, that boosts health and balances hormones. It provides a day-by-day, step-by-step plan for maximizing health via holistic methods and natural health practices that are sure to enliven the body, mind, and spirit with health and vitality. She is a masterful nutritionist and a blessing to those seeking her help."

Jack Tips, PhD

Live Vibrantly! 10 Steps To Maintain Youthfulness, Increase Energy, Restore Your Health

"As a wellness coach and integrated body therapist I can say that Johanna's work is top notch, professional and, best of all, gets results. Her knowledge, caring and depth of understanding of the body, nutrients, and physiology is very impressive. Her coaching me personally has improved my energy, the way I shop, how I treat my body, and definitely taken me to the next level of optimal health. It IS easy and simple; it is NOT a diet or drudgery. I will continue to follow through with her and happily refer my clients."

Warren Angelo, I.B.T, C.W.C

"When I came to see Johanna I had been experiencing menopausal bloat and "brain fog." Her nutritional and lifestyle recommendations were easy to follow. Within 4 weeks, my symptoms had disappeared, I had lost 8 pounds, and I felt great! I have kept up with these habits and remained energized and balanced. I highly recommend Johanna!"

Jean Sibley

"I found out about the Breeze Through Menopause program via a post on a friend's Facebook page. I am a breast cancer survivor who is in menopause due to the preventative meds I take (tamoxifen) and have struggled with hot flashes and weight gain. I found the program easy to incorporate into my daily life thanks to the shopping lists and recipes. It was extremely helpful having it broken down into breakfast, dinner and lunch each week. During the three weeks I was following the program, my hot flashes decreased and I lost 8 lbs!" Andrea, Summer Breeze Through Menopause Program, 2014

Katarina Köster
Johanna is the most positive person I know and brings that attitude with her into her coaching. Her nutrition teachings are solidly based in what's good for everyone: people, earth, and all living creatures. She

will create a customized nutrition program tailored for individual success, and her positive attitude will make it a fun experience and see you all the way through to a healthier you.

Johanna Thorn is a one-of-a-kind nutritionist! She portrays a high level of sincerity in every task she undertakes. Her comprehensive approach makes her a very unique nutritionist. Johanna offers support far beyond nutrition. She firmly believes in eating right and using the highest quality nutritional supplements available, thereby giving her clients the ability to quickly achieve and maintain their personal health goals and live a happier, healthier and longer life. She is compassionate, patient and beyond encouraging. Through her knowledge, guidance, warmth and positive support, Johanna inspired me to embark upon a lifestyle transformation with nutrition and wellness at its core.

Lily Zukowski

"In the fall of 2011, Johanna's father found out he had colon cancer. We immediately told Jo and she got on to it right away. She came up from California and stayed a month with us. Dec.01, 2011 was our 60th wedding anniversary. Dec.09 Chuck, (her father) had his surgery. All went well. His recovery was so remarkable even with 6 months of chemo. Jo used a combination of food and herbal support for him. All the three doctors involved, the family doctor, the surgeon, the oncologist were amazed. All said ""Whatever you are doing, keep doing it. It works."" Today at 85 he is still cancer free and has amazing energy...Thanks to our caring daughter, Johanna.

I personally have not had good health most of my life, even being told I have MS. Last summer I started having stomach troubles. I ate Tums and other things to no avail but didn't tell Jo. I had been on prescription painkillers for a few years. Finally the family doctor said I should stop as my kidneys were slowing down. I had acid reflux, irritable bowel syndrome and was down to 85 pounds from 112 pounds.

Now Jo took over. Again she used a combination of food and herbal support. She also encouraged acupuncture and massage which I started doing weekly.

As of this time in July 2015 I am up to 91 pounds, introducing more and more foods into my diet and feeling so much better. My kidney values on recent lab work showed improvement from 51-70 in just one month. Our family doctor could not believe it. Very impressed with Johanna he is. Again he said "Whatever you are doing, keep it up. It works."

Thank you my dear Johanna.

Love,

Mom

(Irene Thorn)

Live Vibrantly! 10 Steps To Maintain Youthfulness, Increase Energy, Restore Your Health

By Johanna Thorn, N.C.

Of

I Live Vibrantly

Live Vibrantly! 10 Steps To Maintain Youthfulness, Increase
Energy, Restore Your Health

Copyright © 2014 Johanna Thorn

All rights reserved. No portion of the book may be reproduced or
utilized in any form or by any means, electronic or mechanical,
including photocopying, recording, or by any other information
storage and retrieval system, without permission from Author.

Printed in the United States of America

First Printing, 2015

Johanna Thorn
4152 Meridian St. Ste.105359
Bellingham, WA
98226

www.iLiveVibrantly.com

May this book support you, guide you and teach you how to launch your life beyond the ordinary, beyond your excuses, beyond your boundaries and into vibrant realms. May you enjoy a life filled with all the joy, health and love you could possibly endure. A life with no regrets, filled with laughter and fun. Your vibrancy is a reflection of your inner health. Be present, be in the moment. Play, learn, live a long and vibrancy-filled adventure.

Live Vibrantly! 10 Steps to Maintain Youthfu[l] Increase Energy, Restore Your Health

Introduction

. .ɔɔk better, love better, live better.

ᴜᴋe many, even if you do not experience severe health issues, you just know there's room for you to feel better overall. You want to look vibrantly alive; maybe lose or gain a few pounds, strengthen your body and immune system, have more vibrant skin and hair or whatever your desires might be. You could have more energy to do the things you love and to spend with the ones you love, love/like yourself just a little more and live the life you dream of and know can truly be yours. You know there's a better way than worrying that your body is about to betray you at any given moment. You truly believe that it is your, and all of humankind's, birthright to live in harmony with your body and experience joy, pleasure, and vibrant wellness on a daily basis as your reality, that you can thrive agelessly and with vitality.

You're busy, time is precious, and it's not to be wasted. You want to thrive but not if it takes too much effort because your energy really doesn't extend that far and neither does your time. You're confused by all the choices out there that are supposed to support your health and don't even know where to begin or what choices are really the best for you.

You can start your future starting today by adopting the *Live Vibrantly* 10 step blueprint which will support and enable you to flourish physically, mentally, emotionally and spiritually.

Live Vibrantly! 10 Steps To Maintain Youthfulness, Increase Energy, Restore Your Health

This is why I have written this simple introduction to the 10 step blueprint — to act as your guide and support you to define and design what living vibrantly is for you and your family, so at the end of the day you all get to say, "I Live Vibrantly!" Even just saying that puts your mind and body in a different mindset; with its positive affirmation you begin your journey.

The *Live Vibrantly* 10 step blueprint is not just another diet, paleo, traditional or nutrition book. It is a unique combination of principles and a way of living that promotes and sustains high levels of vibrancy in those who practice them. In this book I have broken down the fundamentals of what it takes to begin upping your vibrancy levels. First we will explore the 10 steps of the *Live Vibrantly* blueprint, how they work, why, and how you can make them your own.

Next we will look at how food supports you, how to stock your pantry, and how to shop. A special treat includes a shopping list template and three-day sample menu plus implementation guide.

As mentioned, there is so much more to living at your highest vibrancy on a daily basis than just food. Though food is your foundation, many other pieces make up the entire circle. How much you move every day, the products you use in your home and on your body, what you think and what you feel are all elements that complete your circle. How do you pull all the pieces together? This is your guidebook. If you have specific health issues the blueprint contained here can lay the foundation for your healing. There are notes when a certain practice should not be undertaken by individuals with certain health challenges.

You are a bio-unique individual. There is only one version of you and I know you want it to be the best possible version ever. What works for your neighbor, your best friend, or another family member may not work for you. For this reason, in my one-on-one coaching we go deep, all the way to your cellular matrix and work at that level. That being said, the guidelines and principles outlined here in this book are what I use in that work and lay the foundation for you to take yourself to the next level. With basic guidelines and choices you test and define what works for you. Remembering that life is not stagnant, every day you will make different choices that support you where you are in each moment. Knowing what those choices are is the key. You move at your own pace. Within these pages you will discover the pieces you need to take your life to that vibrant level you know exists within you, and to maintain it and sustain it once you get there. It will become your life, what you do without even having to think about it. Initially starting this journey will require some thought process and the intent is to get you to that place where you just know and do, without much time spent deliberating.

Don't overthink things, stress or obsess over any of it at any time or stage; just do the best you can at each given moment and circumstance. You are learning how to make the best choices for you. You are learning how to live a vibrant harmonious lifestyle that will serve you, your loved ones, your environment, the planet and its population. Have FUN with it and yourself. Eating and living vibrantly should be pleasurable rituals and joyful moments, not pain-filled, torturous ones.

Live Vibrantly! 10 Steps To Maintain Youthfulness, Increase Energy, Restore Your Health

Why Listen To Me?

I was born two months premature and was deemed a "sickly" child. Continually, I suffered from severe allergies, infection upon infection, digestive issues, bronchial/lung issues, among many, many other things. These all got progressively worse as I got older. I became curious about nutrition and its effect on quality of life at the age of 13 upon visiting a naturopathic doctor for the first time in Toronto, Ontario, Canada. He introduced me to a rotation diet and natural health food stores to help cope with allergies after doing testing to figure those out. Come to find I was allergic to almost everything! Putting his advice into practice helped and I was intrigued by how different I felt when I applied his teachings and when I didn't. My health issues all came together at the age of 22 when a diagnosis of Chronic Fatigue Syndrome was presented. The doctors told me that I would have to live with my debilitating symptoms for the rest of my life and learn ways to "manage" them as best I could.

My reaction to that? "Unacceptable!" There had to be a way back to health. Some respite had been gained from the severity of my symptoms in the past by using the rotation diet, so I knew food was connected to how bad or how good I felt. Through my own research and trial and error, a nutrition program evolved that eventually brought me out of that state of dis-ease and into the best health to date I had ever experienced.

That took over three years from the day of diagnosis. I was happy but still anxious that the symptoms would return at any time. I knew I needed to learn how to live in harmony with my body, not in fear of it.

That anxiety stayed with me and a high-stress lifestyle led to other health issues which pushed me into a very early menopause and for the next several years my health deteriorated gradually, and included systemic Candida overgrowth (fungal/yeast overgrowth within the body). I lived in fear, but I pushed on as I firmly believed a higher vibrancy of living could be mine, I just had to figure out how to get there. I searched and researched, looking for ways to bring my hormones and body back to a place of balance and thriving instead of struggling. I made huge leaps forward as I learned but it seemed nothing could permanently get rid of the Candida and bring hormonal balance. At that point I discovered I could deepen my knowledge and turn my passion for seeking nutrition knowledge into preventing others from suffering as I had. That marked the beginning of a journey and quest that led to Bauman College in 2000, where I earned a nutrition consultant certification. In 2001 I had the great privilege and blessing of being introduced to world-renowned teacher and author Dr. Jack Tips, Ph.D., C.C.N, C.Hom. Through Dr. Tips I was introduced to the work and teachings of "Doc" A.S. Wheelwright which changed the way I understood and approached nutrition. It is Doc's teachings that are a huge part of the foundational principles that make up the *Live Vibrantly* 10 step blueprint.

Not only did I learn how to support others, but I also learned how to take my own quality of life up many notches to the level of vibrancy I had always believed existed. (Yes, I was able to reverse the early menopause and bring my hormones back to a place of balance and bring my body out of its candida-riddled state!) For the first time ever I never feared a relapse of Chronic Fatigue Syndrome or any other symptoms, ever again! Why? Because I had begun to learn how to support and live in harmony with my body on all levels physically, mentally, and emotionally. For the first time the fear was gone.

I had been alive up until then. At 32, I began living, and now as I practice what I have learned and continue to learn, I get to live vibrantly every day. I had created a second chance for myself to FLOURISH. This is my wish for all; that YOU may flourish, and so I have made this my career! And over the years as I have supported many others to reach that level of vibrantly flourishing, my true joy and service has been found.

What Do You Stand To Gain?

Better health, better sleep, better life, better you. More energy, more vibrancy, more you.

My mission is to show you how simple, economical and not labor intensive living the *Live Vibrantly* way of life can truly be. My greatest reward and gift is when people share with me how what we co-created together has improved their quality of life and enjoyment of it. It has supported them to lose weight or heal a health issue, given them their joy of life back and their youthfulness, and taken away that fear that their body would give out on them at any moment. It has given them the freedom to be that vibrant living soul they always believed in.

Perfection is not the goal here, nor does it exist, by the way. That is the opposite of what the *Live Vibrantly* blueprint is all about. Moderation is key; there is no room for extreme anything. Don't attempt all of this at once. Pick one place, one piece and start there. Find the one that resonates the most with you. Make that shift. Notice how you feel, how you think, how you move, how you sleep, how you smell (I know that sounds kind of weird but trust me, after you begin to make changes you will understand why I ask you to notice this) after making this change. Get to know this tiny new piece of you. Have fun together.

Then you'll be ready to move on to the next piece. You don't have to follow this book from beginning to end if that doesn't feel right for you. Jump around if that's what suits you. Randomly pick things if that's what works for you. Work your way through all the pieces as you wish and at your pace. After all, it is about finding your bio-uniqueness along the way and supporting that to thrive and flourish vibrantly.

Live Vibrantly! 10 Steps To Maintain Youthfulness, Increase Energy, Restore Your Health

Now before you move into the actual *Live Vibrantly* 10 step blueprint, go to the journaling pages and answer the before you begin questions. These will help you get clear on what you wish to get out of this book and how to use it in your life.

"Wondering how to turn this 10 Step Blueprint into your life? Go to: http://ilivevibrantly.com/programs/live-vibrantly-series/
There you will find the Live Vibrantly! 21 Day Reset To Maintain Youthfulness, Increase Energy, Restore Your Health online program. 21 Days where I walk you through transforming your life step by step. Your vibrant self awaits you. Start your journey now. Go to: http://ilivevibrantly.com/programs/live-vibrantly-series/ to find out how."

Part 1:

Live Vibrantly! 10 Step Blueprint

Following are the 10 basic steps to the *Live Vibrantly* way of life, broken down for you.

1. *EAT: a <u>variety</u> of organic plants, vegetables, seeds, nuts, and fruit – both raw and cooked. Include herbs and spices in small amounts; again moderation.; otherwise these herbs and spices can become therapeutic.*

   What does that mean, exactly? It means that every meal you eat should include some form of plant matter, vegetables, in both raw and cooked combinations. Plant based foods should be the foundation of your plate. Additionally one meal a day could include A) a small quantity of seeds or nuts that have been soaked, fermented and sprouted and B) a small quantity of herbs and spices, either dried or fresh.

2. *EAT: pasture-raised, wild-caught sustainable animal proteins in small amounts – both raw and cooked*

   There is a place for grass-fed, pasture-raised sourced butters, cheeses, eggs, offal and meats in our diets. This can be a controversial subject — the including of animal proteins in one's diet. I believe that small amounts eaten responsibly, sourced from responsible, sustainable sources, have a place. If you just cannot get on board with this thought then you can skip this step but know that the latest science and research shows that vegan/vegetarian diets are deficient in their amino acid profiles/proteins such as methionine, vitamins such as B12/folate, A, D and K. (<u>PubMed study</u>) These are essential for optimal health and function. I know we can all agree, though, that the process of commercial farming, hormone fed, antibiotic-filled animals raised in inhumane environments is unacceptable.

3. *EAT: small amounts of traditionally fermented foods at every meal*

Why? The bacteria from fermented foods feed our good bacteria and keep them happy. They help reestablish the ecosystem of the·bacteria that support your gut health and starve the bacteria that promote inflammation and opportunistic invaders. Beware though; not all fermented foods are equal! It's important to save vinegar fermented foods for special occasions and focus more on traditional ferments. (Note: if you have a Candida overgrowth issue then this might not be a step for you yet; some people with Candida can tolerate the fermented foods and it helps – others cannot.)

4. *DRINK: pure, clean water; filtered best*

Clean, pure water is the only water that will allow you to thrive and sustain you at high vibrancy levels. These days there is everything from toxic chemicals, to drugs or parasites in our water. A good filtration system will help remove most of these. Water from plastic bottles and irresponsibly sourced water should be avoided. The plastics end up leaching into the water, causing hormone disruption and many other health issues. Irresponsibly sourced is, well, what it is and should be avoided if at all possible.

5. *FAST: Don't eat continuously, allow yourself to feel hungry between meals; fast one day a week*

You may or may not be familiar with this concept and I will be going into further detail about it in my next book. Your digestion is best supported by allowing it to "empty out" between meals and one day a week. If you have severe digestive issues this step is not for you yet. This one-day fast can consist of just juicing, just bone broth or a combination of both to get you started with the concept. According to our body cycles, Friday is the best day of the week for this in case you wanted to know that, but you can pick any day that works for you. Fasting means dinner the night before is your last meal until breakfast the day after you eat nothing. Full-day fasting may or may not be for you at this stage.

6. *MOVE; everyday, somehow, someway for at least 10 – 20 minutes*

Stagnant pools of water become a breeding ground for the wrong kind of bacteria; NOT the life-promoting kind. Your body is the pool; keep the water moving! This does not have to involve strenuous exercise, especially if you have been sedentary for a long time. Just move! Park a little further away when you go to the store, take the stairs instead of the elevator, walk somewhere instead of drive. You get the idea. Then build it up from there.

7. *SUN: expose yourself to real sunlight/daylight without sunscreen 20 minutes a day*

This is my favorite and further detail about this is in the lifestyle section of this book. For me there is nothing like the feel of warm sun on my face and skin that soothes and relaxes me. That feeling makes me smile every time. Enjoy the feeling, smile into your heart; it will thank you too. (While you're doing this is a good time to practice your breathing, too.)

8. *BREATHE: stop periodically throughout the day and take 3 – 5 deep belly breaths, especially before you eat*

Many individuals practically run through their days with no idea of time passing or how it got to be the end of the day, or else they struggle to make it to the end of the day. They do not recall eating or notice how they feel except when feeling bad. These fast-paced, high-stress days keep you in flight or fight mode. This is not supportive to high vibrancy and health. You want to be in relaxed mode as much as you can and especially when about to eat. STOP. BREATHE. NOTICE.

9. *SLEEP: deep, refreshing, restorative, uninterrupted sleep*

There is nothing that can restore your vitality like deep, solid, uninterrupted sleep. Create ways to make this happen for you as much as possible. Sometimes there are circumstances that do not allow for this but know that your health will suffer over time with continued lack of sleep.

10. *LOVE: come from a place of love in all you do; for yourself, for others*

Ahhh, the ultimate — love. If you come from a place of love for yourself, and I mean true, authentic love that accepts you as a whole for who you are in this present moment, the pretty and the not so pretty parts of you, then you are well on your way to upping your vibrancy levels and living vibrantly every day! You will automatically take that into all your relationships, tasks, activities. Love usually overrides fear as well and keeps us moving on that path that is our adventure called life.

How It Works

When you examine and sample the recipes you may notice a theme running through all of them. The foods have been combined to maximize nutrition, make it bioavailable (the degree to which food nutrients are available for absorption and utilization in the body) and put less stress on your digestive system, thus supporting your microbiomes (the microorganisms in a particular environment including the body or a part of the body).

The basic formula for how to best combine your foods comes from information and research that I was truly blessed to come upon some fourteen years ago. Many of you may not have heard of the life and work of "Doc" A.S. Wheelwright, a genius of a man and healer so ahead of his time. The principles he learned and taught about food combining (not what you are probably familiar with) were passed down to me by my dear friend, colleague, teacher, and mentor, Dr. Jack Tips, who worked directly with Doc Wheelwright for six years. Dr. Tips wrote The ProVita plan back in 1992 and the information in there changed my life and the lives of the people I have coached and worked with ever since. And the most astounding thing?! The information in that book is still pertinent today and publicly science is only now beginning to catch up. That is usually unheard of in the world of nutrition! As you may have noticed, information will be released and perpetuated only to be found "out of date" several years later. Later this year (2015) a new nutrition book using the ProVita foundation, coauthored by Dr. Tips and myself, will be released.

For now, let's just recap what "Doc" taught as the formula and some of the main principles behind these habits.

The basic formula is the 5+5 principle. The focus for this formula is on proteins and vegetables; ALWAYS eat vegetables combined with your protein. Vegetables are essential in order to process proteins from start to finish. And with one cooked protein you eat four raw proteins. (see list of proteins in Resources)

This ensures a complete amino acid profile within your meal so your body will not be robbing amino acids from your organs to digest your meal. With one cooked vegetable, you eat four raw vegetables. This also ensures you get the RNA/DNA factors from your vegetables and the differing nutrient profiles from the food in both its raw and cooked version. Lightly cooked vegetables provide inner cell (chromatin) factors rich in DNA and RNA which are the building blocks of body revitalization. These factors are missed or in short supply if you exist solely on raw or fermented vegetables because most of us cannot break down the indigestible cellulose to get the chromatin factors from the raw version. That is pretty much a direct quote from Dr. Jack Tips, helping to explain this little discussed and taught principle. For many of you I know this is the first time you have even heard of this 5+5 formula. Don't overthink it, it's really quite simple.

Why It Works

So what this breaks down to and means is that some cooked vegetables are more nutritious to you at a cellular level than in their raw state. The heat of cooking breaks down the thick cell walls of the plants and enables your body to absorb their nutrients better, therefore making them bioavailable. However, this primarily applies to steaming/sautéing vegetables, the key being in "lightly" cooking. Lightly roasting also works as it seals in the nutrients and the vegetables are still crisp inside. Slow cooked at low temperature vegetables are also good as there is a liquid medium needed for this type of cooking and the nutrients also cook down into that liquid, making it a concentrated nutritious part of the meal.

For example, steamed carrots have a higher content of beta carotene than their raw counterpart. Use the steam liquid in a soup or sauce base. Using traditional methods to ferment them takes them to another level and adds the beneficial bacteria the body needs so badly as well. It is best to not only eat a variety of food but to use a variety of non-cooking, cooking and preserving methods.

Be sure to add some healthy fat and something fermented (not necessarily alcoholic just in case you were heading in that direction) to this 5+5 meal combination and you are all set. Benefits of eating this way include but are not limited to more energy, sharper brain, happy microbiomes, happy digestive system, less toxic stress, stronger immune system, automatic weight control/balance, better sleep, and balanced hormones.

For these reasons, I resource and create recipes that could be categorized as raw, vegan, vegetarian, traditional, paleo, or gluten free, just to name a few. Personally, I don't like to label recipes that way, though I know some of you find that helpful. I just call my style the *Live Vibrantly* lifestyle and way. I love to create my own recipes and there are also so many amazing recipes already out there so why not mix and share? No boredom or ruts justified, too many resources for that. In the resources section I have included the resources I go to for inspiration and ideas, and most of the recipes here, unless otherwise noted, come from me or have been adapted by me to meet the 5+5 formula and could have been originally inspired by someone else's recipe.

How To Make It Yours

I take recipes that I see and rearrange them, add to them, or take away from them, in order to make the nutrients more bioavailable (by using the 5+5 formula as the foundation) and use what's available per season. For example, in winter there is less raw food and I make use of soups, sea vegetables, root vegetables, micro greens and sprouts. In spring, as all that fresh food starts to become abundant again the raw food starts to increase bit by bit until it cumulates in the warmest summer months. Then with late fall and cooler weather I start moving back to more cooked foods, more roots and into the brothier, saucier meals, as I like to refer to them.

This is one of the greatest tools in life I can share with you — how to take anything and turn it into a seasonal *Live Vibrantly* meal, a meal that is bioavailable and feeds you at a cellular level. These habits are the best way to support and keep your microbiomes happy, your brain sharp, up your vibrancy levels and live at your highest vibrancy the rest of your life! This way of eating is age defying and makes sure you have all the components to keep your body functioning at its prime. Life = Life. How alive your food is dictates how alive you are. It's that simple.

Here is a copy of my *Live Vibrantly* daily food breakdown and sample chart. Print it and keep it on your fridge for reference and guidance. Soon it will become YOUR habit, YOUR way of doing things, and you won't need to think about it, you'll just be doing it. Keep in mind that this is the basic starting point you will begin working from and as you learn more about your bio-unique self, and to meet life's ever changing requirements, adjustments will happen.

Daily food breakdown:

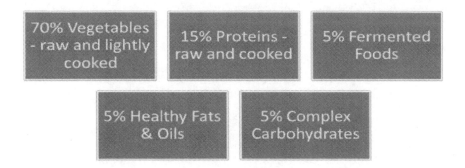

Sample of what your plate looks like at a protein meal using 5+5 formula:

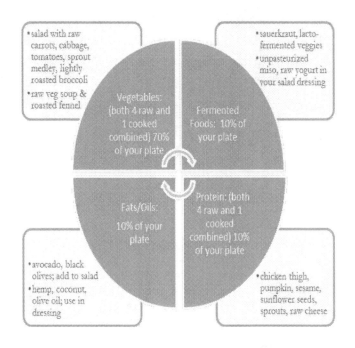

Live Vibrantly! 10 Steps To Maintain Youthfulness, Increase Energy, Restore Your Health

Now before you move into the actual *Live Vibrantly* 10 step blueprint, go to the journaling pages and answer the before you begin questions. These will help you get clear on what you wish to get out of this book and how to use it in your life.

"Wondering how to turn this 10 Step Blueprint into your life? Go to: http://ilivevibrantly.com/programs/live-vibrantly-series/
There you will find the Live Vibrantly! 21 Day Reset To Maintain Youthfulness, Increase Energy, Restore Your Health online program. 21 Days where I walk you through transforming your life step by step. Your vibrant self awaits you. Start your journey now. Go to: http://ilivevibrantly.com/programs/live-vibrantly-series/ to find out how."

Part 2

Food As Foundation

Food is not the end all or be all of your *Live Vibrantly* way of life but it is the foundation of everything else you do and plays a huge role. Why?

Remember? Life = life. How much life is in your food = how much life you will experience. Moderation and variety are the keys to healthy eating.

Food is your main source of nourishment for your physical body. It provides fuel for you to function. What you put into your body as food dictates whether you will move through your day, your life, full of energy, happy, alert, and sharp, or lethargic, struggling, foggy-brained, and cranky. Which would you rather be?

Did you know that the new saying now is not "you are what you eat," it's "you are what your microbiota or bugs eat?" Yes! Our primary focus here will be on your microbiomes and making them happy. Your what??!!

Your microbiomes. You've read that word here several times now and been given a brief definition. But what is it? Simply put; the bugs (bacteria or microbiota) that live in and on us! Okay, I won't go too deeply into the details here, but you do need to know some basics in order to up the vibrancy levels of your life.

Today we hear so much about inflammation and there is hardly anyone who does not experience it in some part of their body in some way. Inflammation is the chief health concern being reported on today in magazines like Time, on local and national news commentaries, on the Internet, and so on. Your microbiomes are the first line of defense against inflammation but has its work cut out for it and struggles because of antibiotics, genetically altered foods, and environmental toxins. Inflammation plays a large role in exacerbating all health issues and symptoms.

Why do you even need these "bugs" on you and in you anyway? Because pathogens keep your immune system vigilant and the beneficial probiotic bacteria keep the pathogens in check — "nature's perfection," to quote a colleague of mine who put it eloquently.

The microbiomes are finally gaining more notice in the field of nutrition science and even in mainstream media. Working to rebalance my own health issues over the years was how I discovered that my microbiomes played a major role in that success and it's a topic I happen to find very exciting and fascinating. As researchers delve deeper into this incredible microscopic world, they're finding connections between having happy bacteria in your bellies and having a happy, healthy life! Now that's quite a profound statement. Basically your body and your "bugs," when in balance, are working together for the same desired outcome.

One key connection I would like to point out here that will help you understand why I'm going on and on about "bugs," is that your microbiomes can cause your brain to experience things like increased anxiety or calm, increased learning, enhanced memory and various moods depending on the ratio of beneficial bacteria to pathogens. And on the flip side, your brains can alter the microbiome through hormones and neurotransmitters such as serotonin, dopamine and cortisol, just to name a few. The good news is you can support your brain to be sharper with the right food choices such as those outlined in the *Live Vibrantly* 10 step blueprint. You can support hormones and neurotransmitters with the same beneficial food choices, and you can support both with positive mental thought. The *Live Vibrantly* 10 step blueprint shows you how.

Celiac, leaky gut, dysbiosis, in fact all digestive issues, are in part connected to your microbiome balance. Autoimmune issues are also connected to microbiome balance. We won't be going into detail here, though, because that's another discussion. I just wanted to mention it here in case you have been diagnosed with any of these digestive imbalances or an auto-immune issue, you would know that the 10 step blueprint will help to support balance and healing for you.

Some fun facts about your microbiomes:

- Your microbiomes are unique to your genetics; it's your personal, biochemically-individual microbiome.
- Your microbiomes can control your thoughts, feelings and <u>food cravings</u>; ever wonder why even though you try to make healthy changes the cravings still won't go away?
- Your microbiomes have a direct link to the level of autoimmune activity against your thyroid, which translates to your gut is connected to your thyroid health. (According to PubMed, some groups estimate that 27 million Americans have thyroid disease, and about 13 million of them are undiagnosed.)
- Your microbiomes' health influences your health. It's directly related to your hormone health. This includes the brain's leptin receptors (hormone that tells you when we're full or not)

which plays a huge role in your appetite and storage of fat. Yes! Your "bugs" can affect how you lose or gain weight!!!

I hope now you understand why the things we are going to focus on all revolve around supporting your microbiomes, which will allow you to nourish yourself at a cellular level. This is your foundation to *Live Vibrantly!*

The *Live Vibrantly* Kitchen and Pantry

Kitchen Essentials:
High-speed blender
Food processor
Hand grater
Crockpot (best to have a programmable one; they start new around $40 on Amazon. That being said, I'm also still using an older model I already own because I need more than one and it just has high and low settings on it. It works; you just have to be home while it's on.)

Great if you happen to have, but not necessary:
Vegetable juicer
Dehydrator
Spiralizer (for making "pasta" from zucchini and other vegetables)
Mason jars
Citrus juicer
Mixing bowls, glass, different sizes
Whisk
Good sharp knives
Coco-jack (to easily open coconuts; see amazonlist)
Grain grinder

I like to always keep certain fresh ingredients on hand that allow me to make multiple items. I usually buy whatever looks good, is local, in season and/or is on sale. Check the resources page in the bonus section for where you can get some of these items if you have trouble finding them. I am sharing with you what I like to keep on hand in my kitchen so you will start to get a sense of how to always have what you need to create delicious food on the fly. It can be expensive to begin to build your pantry if you don't already have many of these items on hand. I suggest you prioritize the items according to your tastes and needs; then each time you shop purchase one item. Replace items when they are on sale, even before you run out if you can. Buy nonperishable items you use frequently in large quantity; that will save you much in the long run. Sometimes finding a friend to split a large quantity with is also the way to go. Get creative!

I also happen to be the "PostIt queen" but I suggest a notebook to keep all your ideas and creations in. Write things down as you make them so you won't forget for next time. Write next to it how much you (and/or your family members) liked or disliked it so you can adjust next time, make exactly the same, or never again.

Pantry...

Nuts, seeds, superfoods, herbs, spices, and oils are all stored in glass jars. I actually keep my nuts and seeds in the freezer to further prevent oxidation. As soon as I am getting low on a seed or nut that is ready to use and eat, I get a batch soaking and fermenting right away so I don't run out. I also try to have at least three options ready to go at all times. All nuts and seeds require soaking, fermenting and sprouting to break down phytic acid and make their nutrients bioavailable. I soak them overnight in a bowl with 1 cup nut or seed, ¼ cup water kefir, and 3–4 cups filtered (non-chlorinated) water. Nuts like almonds I tend to let sit for a couple more hours in the morning. Next rinse and strain off the water. Let them sit damp to begin the sprouting process before dehydrating —seeds up to 4 hours, nuts up to 8 hours. Then, if you don't have a dehydrator, spread them on a cookie sheet , turn on your oven to 180 degrees or the warm setting and leave them in the oven to dehydrate for about 24 hours or until they are your desired crispness. I don't season mine as I like to grind them into flours and use them for dips and sauces as well as milks.

In my pantry you will always find...

Nuts and Seeds:

- Almonds (preferably not from California which are all flash pasteurized), hazelnuts, cashews, pumpkin seeds, sunflower seeds, sesame seeds both black and tan. I also have walnuts, pecans, pistachios, pine nuts, brazil nuts, chia and flax seeds.

Dried herbs and spices include:

- Thyme, oregano, basil, rosemary, herbs de Provence blend, cumin, ground ginger, turmeric, curry, cinnamon, ground sage, red pepper flakes, chipotle powder, Cajun spice, sea and pink Himalayan salt, black pepper, garlic powder. And my favorite new addition is cardamom.

Oils/Fats are:

- Homemade animal lard or tallow (large quantities should be stored in the freezer but small batches can be left out of refrigeration), raw extra virgin coconut oil, ghee, avocado oil, unfiltered extra virgin olive oil, flax or hemp oil, sesame oil, toasted sesame oil, and one more nut oil. (As nut oils can be expensive, I alternate each time I purchase.)

Vinegars include:

- Unfiltered raw apple cider, coconut, balsamic, rice, red wine, and one "special" one. Right now I have a thyme vinegar from Italy that I am loving.

Superfoods are a great way to add extra nutrition to your meals and day. I love to always keep:

- Raw green powder blend containing e3live, blue green algae, spirulina, maca powder, matcha tea or powder, raw cacao nibs and powder, raw nori sheets, wakame, dulse flakes and strips, goji berries and mulberries.

Miscellaneous items include:

- Wild, line-caught sardines, wild, line-caught anchovies, oysters, caviar, capers, unsweetened shredded or flaked coconut, back-up jar of unpasteurized raw miso, several different kinds of herbal and green teas, nutritional yeast, wheat-free tamari or raw shoyu, raw coconut aminos, raw sprouted tahini butter, raw sprouted nut butters, coconut flour, a couple of sprouted ancient grain flours, sprouted rye flour, dates, pure maple syrup, raw honey, coconut sugar, vermouth (great with seafood!), Madeira (fabulous to cook mushrooms in) and Chinese rice wine.

I always have water kefir going and make "sodas" and fermented veggie blended drinks. As well there is usually a lacto-fermented veggie brewing, raw yogurt or some "experiment" happening. I don't make kombucha at the moment but will be adding it back into the mix shortly. I don't make my own sauerkraut either because I am incredibly blessed to be in contact with others who make beautiful kraut and I love to support them. Look in the resources section for where to buy water kefir grains, kombucha culture and more.

Fridge and Fresh Produce...
Dairy:

- Pastured chicken and/or duck eggs (not fed any grain feed preferably) (not actual dairy but usually found in that section), grass-fed butter; cow or goat, raw, grass-fed cow cheese, hard and soft goat or sheep cheese from Europe (not local because most of the microbes used in the USA are GMO), raw goat milk (raw cow milk also good) (to use in smoothies and to make raw homemade yogurt) plain yogurt, preferably raw. (I like to make my own using the countertop method with raw goat milk when I can get it.)

Vegetables:

- Jalapenos, cucumber —English or Persian my favs —, celery, red and green cabbage (I just have a little piece cut off the head at the store and then stored in a sealed container it lasts for several weeks in fridge), salad greens, fresh basil, oregano, thyme, parsley, cilantro, sprouts and micro greens – several different kinds, preferably at least four varieties — tomatoes, carrots, red bell peppers, mushrooms; whatever is local to you and currently in season

Fruit:

- Apples, lemons (I prefer Meyers), limes, avocados, young coconuts (not really fruit, but usually stocked in fruit area of store); whatever is local and in season

Condiments:

- Onion, garlic, ginger, shallots; whatever is local and in season, grass-fed beef, lamb, pork or pasture chicken bones, chicken or beef livers (really any kind of bones and offal you can get) and chicken feet for your chicken bone broth. (I always have homemade stock/broth on hand.)

I used to have the tiniest kitchen, by the way, and learned you do not need massive quantities of things unless you have a big family to feed. I had little bits of things in great variety. And with these items I could whip up something delicious on the fly at any time for myself or guests; the possibilities are endless. Nor do you need a big, updated modern kitchen to cook fabulous meals; good old-fashioned basics work amazingly well, and they often force you to get very creative.

How To Shop In *Live Vibrantly* Style

The key to shopping is to eat local and in season as much as you can! Many raise the objection that eating healthy is more expensive. Well, in some cases the price tag might be a bit higher (not always though!) but ask yourself this, can you afford the consequences of not making these choices for yourself and your children? The cost of vitality lost, illness or dis-ease is much higher. When I coach my one-on-one clients, one of the things I help with is how to source locally as much as possible. Google your area, find out what's around you. Ask people at Farmers Markets, local health food stores, your friends, neighbors, go for a day drive adventure and pack a picnic, go for a bike ride or a hike while you check things out around you; use your local resources.

A tip I often share with my clients is to frequent your local farmers market(s) or farms and get to know the people. Many use organic practices but are too small to afford the organic certification or don't do it for other reasons. These "little guys" could be more "organic" than massive farms with the certification. Look for farms and farmers using permaculture practices. If they are relatively close by, ask if you can go visit the farm. See how things are done. Develop relationships with the people who produce the food you eat. This can be more significant than any labeling. Sign up for local CSAs; it's not just for boxes of vegetables and fruits anymore. You can often get pasture meats, eggs and other items too. If a box or order is too much food for you, find someone to share it with. Take the time to go see the farm you choose, meet the people, observe their practices, and ask questions. It makes a difference, really. Try to buy as little as possible from stores. Get to know your community, ask around, and you might be happily surprised at what you discover.

Ways To Save Money:

- As mentioned, Farmers Markets offer an exceptional way to spend more of your money on actual food instead of packaging, manufacturing, distributing and so on. In the end you actually get more food for your money. When markets are not an option, look to see what is on sale at your local stores and work your menus to match.

- Freeze, preserve, ferment, or dehydrate items when you buy large quantities on sale. Traditional fermenting helps preserve foods so they keep easily and last longer while providing the bacteria you need to keep your friendly bacteria fed and happy.

- Plant a garden; you don't need much space. If you are short on room, think vertical and pots. Learn how to forage for wild edibles in your area. There are more and more classes being offered about this subject these days.

- Reuse and recycle everything you possibly can — bags, jars, containers and so on. Buy secondhand when it's an option, especially books and kitchen gadgets.

Ways To Save Time in the Kitchen:

Realistically, unless you are like me and love spending hours in the kitchen creating and playing, you want as many time-saving tricks as possible. With the 3-day menu included in this book you begin to get a taste for how to best leverage the time you do spend.

- Cook larger batches of food, more than you need for that one meal. Of course sometimes when trying a new recipe for the first time you want to be sure you're going to like it first before you start making big batches of it, which is why many of my recipes only serve 2 and do well when doubled.

- Stock up on your staples when they are on sale, especially non-perishable items. Go in with your friends and neighbors on cases as most stores will give you a discount on such.

- Make, serve and store your food in as few vessels as possible. Blend dressings, sauces, dips with a hand blender right in the container you are going to store it in. I serve food right out of the glass container I'm storing it in. Snap the lid onto the leftovers and you are all set. Less items to wash, less water used.

- Organize your fridge, keep it clean. This makes finding things and using them so much easier. I like to keep all my animal products on the bottom shelves and like with like. So all raw meat stays together, all cooked together, all dairy, all veggies, all fruit, all condiments and so on. This actually saves time because I know what's in my fridge and don't have to look. Saves energy too as the door is not left open forever while I'm searching for something.

- Keep your workspace, no matter how big or small, organized and ready to use at all times. When you are about to make something, gather all your ingredients, wash what needs washing, make sure you have all the equipment you will need ready to go. Pre-measure and pour your ingredients into little dishes or bowls so it's all ready to go if that helps you too. That way putting your food together and creating your dishes will be much easier. Work like a professional chef!

- I also like to keep my juicing/soup container and compost container open and ready to fill so I can just drop things in there as I go. The juicing/soup container is where I put all the items that can be used in juice or added to a broth rather than straight to the compost pile. Examples of these items could be fennel tops, carrot tops, radish tops, beet stems, kale ribs and so much more.

- Plan one meal a week as a "no cook" meal. Instead you use the extra portions you made in creative ways.

I have put together a shopping list template for you if you wish to use it. You can check it out in the Resources section.

You will find a variety of cooked and raw foods combined in the 3 Day Sample Menu that begin to introduce you to how to combine your foods for optimal nutrition to meet your body's needs for the season, and are easy to prepare and require little cleanup time. Let's face it, time is of the essence. I congratulate you on taking this step, making the commitment to creating freedom for yourself to have vibrant health and Live Vibrantly. My wish is for you to have fun doing this and discover easy, new habits. I have created this little 3-day menu as a taste for you and your family. Have everyone participate in preparing the food and make it a family affair! Everyone stands to gain.

Breakfast – The Most Important Meal Of The Day

A little saying I learned a long time ago and like to share with my clients is to eat breakfast like a king, lunch like a prince and dinner like a pauper. We need the most fuel in the morning to get us through the day. Early in the day is when the protein digestive enzymes are at their strongest and eating protein early in the day makes it available when we need it the most, while we are awake and demanding the most of ourselves. This also is when we most need the amino acids from protein to supply serotonin and tryptophan especially to our brains for sustained energy, better moods and rejuvenating sleep at night. If you miss out on breakfast you cannot make up your amino acid loss later in the day; that opportunity is gone.

Breakfast should include a combination of protein, fat and carbohydrates that will fuel you for the day. Ideally, it should be eaten within one hour of waking or by 11 am, whichever works best for you. Many people say they aren't hungry in the morning, but know that this could be one indication of thyroid imbalance. If you are one of those for whom eating breakfast is hard, then eat when you are hungry. You will notice yourself starting to feel hungry in the mornings again once your microbiome and other health issues become balanced.

Lunch – The Meal That Builds On Breakfast And Keeps Us Going Until Night

If at lunch we are to eat as a prince then our lunch portion should be smaller than breakfast but bigger than our dinner portion. I know this is not the norm for many people and could take some getting used to.

Often eating while working at your desk, standing at the kitchen counter or running that errand, oblivious to the fact you are just inhaling food, or skipping lunch entirely to get a project completed, get the laundry in or meet a deadline while munching on anything on hand, has unfortunately taken over the habit of stopping and taking time to eat. Chew your food well. Yes you may only have a few minutes for lunch but doesn't it make so much more sense to eat a smaller quantity of healthy food, eaten properly, recognized and digested by the body so the nutrients actually get to you and fuel you for the rest of the day in both body and mind? As opposed to the other option of inhaling large quantities of whatever and wondering why you feel so uncomfortable, sleepy, ready for a nap and unmotivated, brain dead.

As I mentioned, I like to use extra portions from previous meals put together in new ways for lunch with a couple of new items. Eating out on occasion is fun, especially when it's with other people. Lunch should be consumed by 2 pm in order to work with our body's natural cycle and assimilate your food best. Trying to eat outside, or going for a walk around the block after eating, is a welcome break from the usual indoor environment. Weather permitting, maybe find a patio, park bench, spot on some grass, or even your yard. If you are blessed with being able to get outside to eat lunch then do it!

Dinner – The Meal That Prepares You For Cleansing And Rebuilding

Recalling our little saying at the beginning, we should eat dinner as a pauper. And you're thinking to yourself, what in the world does that mean? Well, it means that dinner should be a lighter meal, especially in quantity of food or portion size. When our bodies are getting the nutrients they need, decreased appetite is an automatic happening. As your day comes to a close and starts preparing for the night's repair and rest ahead, so should we.

Often when making dinner, I like to prepare extra food that I can use for other meals. Other times I will take a couple of hours on Saturday or Sunday and prepare my food for the week. Whatever works for you, the main objective is to prepare your own homemade food the majority of the time and make it easy to put together tasty, quick meals. While we're talking about cooking batches ahead of time and at certain times, I'm going to add a note here too about fermenting and soaking nuts, seeds, flours, lacto-fermented veggies, water kefir, kombucha and whatever other "experiments" you decide to take on. Know that though these things sound like they are huge time commitments and laborious, they are NOT. Most times it takes 5–10 minutes to get something ready to sit overnight and 10-15 minutes on the other end to "finish" it. Some things require a quick 3–5 minutes here or there until it is ready. That's it! It's just getting into the habit and that takes some time and work and I encourage you to persevere as it is so worth it. I like to put my "breads" and flours to soak on Thursday late afternoon as I know Saturday I will be cooking and have time to bake them.

The following recipes contain a variety of nutrients, proteins, fats, fermented food, carbohydrates and fiber.

Please for the sake of a happy microbiome do **NOT** drink coffee or black tea on a regular basis. Instead drink green teas, matcha, herbal teas, fresh young coconut water and milk, fresh vegetable juices, fermented drinks (better on an empty stomach) such as kombucha and water kefir based drinks in 2–4 oz portions at a time. These should be the only beverages besides water (filtered best) that you drink on a regular basis. Note that the emphasis is on regular or daily habits. This is what we are talking about here. There are those special occasions and not so frequent times where a cup of fair trade, organic coffee or fabulous Earl Grey tea or whatever you choose are what you indulge in. Save these things as special treats; you'll enjoy them that much more.

3-Day *Live Vibrantly* Sample Menu and Shopping List

3 Day Sample Menu

Day 1

- Prepare ahead for Day 1: prepare your smoothie ingredients or cereal ingredients depending on which you are having and the lunch soup can be made ahead and kept in the fridge overnight
- Breakfast – BYO Smoothie, Ready to Rock My Day Shake or Chia Power Me Up Cereal
- Lunch – Delightfully Raw Red Pepper Soup
- Dinner – My Taste Buds Are Alive Chimichurri Steak, Steamin' Peas and Rocket Salad

Day 2

- Prepare ahead for Day 2: soak wild rice and prepare the extra steak for lunch tacos
- Breakfast – Perfect Poached Eggs on Sautéed Spinach with Sprout Medley
- Lunch – Steak Tacos with Cauliflower Tortillas
- Dinner – Savory Wild Rice, Microgreen Medley and Braised Radicchio with Balsamic Vinaigrette

Day 3

- Prepare ahead for Day 3: make pistachio pesto for lunch, assemble wraps for grab n go if making ahead
- Breakfast – Wild Rice Hash Bowl
- Lunch – Scrumptious Pistachio Pesto Wraps with Braised Radicchio
- Dinner – "Spaghetti" with Heirloom Marinara or Meat Sauce and Basic Seasonal Salad

Bonus staple recipes: bone broth, basic dressing, cauliflower tortillas, herbed almond crackers, fresh coconut milk

You will need to make the bone broth, cauliflower tortillas and herbed crackers ahead of time for these three days. Recipes can be found in the <u>Foundational Recipe section</u>. The ingredients needed have been included in the shopping list for this 3 day sample menu. Have fun!

Day 1
Breakfast:
BYO *Live Vibrantly* smoothie:
<u>Base:</u>   Young coconut water, filtered water, green tea or matcha powder added to the smoothie with filtered water, raw cow or raw goat milk, nut milk, fresh coconut milk (not from a box and preferably not from a can), bone broth

<u>Protein additions:</u>   (choose any 2–3 of these) raw egg yolk, young coconut meat, almonds, cashews, hazelnuts, walnuts, sesame seeds, hemp seeds, pumpkin seeds, sunflower seeds, flax or chia seeds*, nut/seed butters, plain whole yogurt, fresh liquid whey
*No more than ¼ cup of nuts or seeds and should be soaked, fermented and sprouted first except for flax and chia seeds

<u>Essential fat additions:</u> (choose 1-2, keep to 1 tablespoon max each) coconut oil or coconut butter, flax oil, hemp oil, grass-fed butter, grass-fed ghee, ½ avocado

<u>Greens:</u>   use sprouts (any kind or blend) plus 1-2 other choices, including micro greens (any blend), romaine, spinach, kale, chard,

lettuces or any of your favorite leafy greens and don't forget fresh herbs can go in this category too

Superfoods: (choose any 2–3 of these) raw green powder blend, spirulina, blue-green algae, dulse flakes, wheatgrass, barley grass, maca powder, raw cacao powder, goji berries (just to name a few)

Sweetener: (if absolutely necessary) 1–2 pitted dates, or ½-1 teaspoon of raw honey or pure maple syrup

Get creative!

Tip: the addition of cilantro or basil works well with many of these combinations.

Ready to Rock My Day Shake
Serves 1

> 1 raw egg yolk or 1 tablespoon ground flaxseed or 1 tablespoon soaked, fermented, sprouted almonds, sunflower seeds, or your favorite(s)
>
> ¼ cup sprouts or micro greens – any mix of varieties but try to use at least 4 varieties
>
> 1 cup seasonal leafy greens, torn, lightly packed about 1-2 large leaves or equivalent
>
> 4-6 large fresh basil leaves or ½ teaspoon dry
>
> ¼ cup avocado, about ¼ of a whole (optional)
>
> 1 tablespoon coconut oil (use if not using avocado)
>
> 1 tablespoon grass-fed butter, melted (optional, use especially if not using avocado or coconut oil)
>
> 1 tablespoon chia seeds

½-1 teaspoon spirulina (if you are not used to the taste of spirulina, start with ¼ teaspoon)

½ tablespoon plain whole cow, goat or sheep yogurt (optional)

Pinch of dulse flakes

1 cup bone broth <u>or</u> 1 cup raw milk <u>or</u> filtered water

Place all ingredients in your high-speed blender and blend until smooth.

Note: Everyone's taste buds are different, which is why there are several options and choices within this recipe. Pick the combinations that appeal to you, and experiment. You are going to like some combinations better than others.

Quick tip: Make this the night before and put it in a thermos, store in the fridge overnight, and it will be ready to grab 'n' go in the morning. Drink within 30 minutes of removing thermos from fridge.

Chia Power Me Up Cereal

Serves 2

1 whole young coconut

1 cup chia seeds

½ cup hemp seeds

1 tablespoon raw cacao powder

½-1 teaspoon raw honey

2 tablespoons coconut butter, liquefied (can substitute coconut oil here too)

½ teaspoon cinnamon (for a special treat try ¼ teaspoon ground cardamom in place of cinnamon)

¼ teaspoon spirulina

½ teaspoon maca (optional but highly recommended)

¼ cup sprout medley (mild-flavored ones best)

Pinch of coarse sea or pink Himalayan salt

Cut open the coconut and pour the water into a blender. Scoop the flesh out and add it to the blender. Do remove any of the husk still attached to the flesh before adding it, though. Blend this until it is creamy. Add the raw honey and the rest of the ingredients except the chia and hemp seeds to the blender; blend until mixed well. Split the chia seeds along with the hemp seeds, between two bowls. Pour half the milk mixture over the seed mixture in one bowl and whisk together. Repeat for the other bowl and leave them to thicken for 10–15 minutes. You can leave it overnight for a real porridge feel. You can also warm it on low heat but do **not** make it bubble and boil; you'll start breaking down all the healthy antioxidants and omega 3s. Chew well and enjoy!

Lunch:

Delightfully Raw Red Pepper Soup

Serves 1-2 (can be doubled)

1 cup red bell pepper, diced, about 1 whole

½ cup sprouts or micro greens, any type, preferably a blend of three or more varieties

¼ cup soaked, fermented, sprouted cashews or walnuts

½ cup avocado, about ½ a whole

1 tablespoon lemon juice

1 tablespoon unpasteurized miso, any "flavor"

1 teaspoon fresh basil, about 3 leaves

1 teaspoon dulse flakes

¼-½ teaspoon chipotle, to taste

½ teaspoon fresh dill, chopped, or ¼ teaspoon dried, as garnish (optional)

Blend all ingredients in high-speed blender until smooth. Pour into lunch container and refrigerate.

Note: You can warm this soup, (do not boil as this will destroy the nutrients) if that is your preference, on low temperature.

As an example of how to adapt recipes according to your needs you can also lightly roast the red pepper first, let it cool to room temperature then make the soup as outlined here. I highly recommend this option for those who have trouble digesting raw foods.

Optional: Serve with the herbed almond crackers you made in the prep ahead section and/or some wild line-caught sardines

Dinner:
Make the Chimichurri sauce first, then put the peas on and assemble the salad minus olive oil and lemon. Put the steak on. Finish the peas and dress the salad while the steak is resting. Serve all of it immediately.

Steamin' peas...
Serves 2 (double the recipe if needed so you will have some leftovers to keep for the next few days)

      1 pound fresh peas (okay to substitute with frozen)
      1 tablespoon fresh lemon juice (Meyer lemons best)
      2 tablespoons butter
      1 teaspoon garlic, chopped (optional)

¼-½ teaspoon of cumin (optional) (If you love cumin, use the ½ teaspoon.)

Pinch of salt and fresh cracked pepper to taste

Steam peas for a few minutes until they turn bright green and tender, usually between 2-5 minutes. Transfer to a serving bowl, pour lemon over and toss to coat evenly. Add butter and let melt, toss to coat evenly. Add rest of ingredients and toss to coat evenly. Serve immediately.

Rocket salad...

Serves 2

3 cups of rocket (arugula)

½ cup microgreen medley of at least 4 varieties (sprouts can be substituted)

1 tablespoon Meyer lemon juice (okay to sub regular lemons but not as flavorful)

¼ cup olive oil

1 tablespoon pine nuts (optional but really add to the overall flavor of this salad)

1 tablespoon parmesan or Pecorino Romano shaved or grated (optional)

Sea salt and fresh cracked pepper to taste

Place salad ingredients in a bowl and toss with olive oil and lemon juice. Dust with sea salt and fresh cracked pepper.

My Taste Buds Are Alive Chimichurri Steak

Chimichurri Sauce

(Note: This sauce is great with eggs or in wraps/rolls too; use your imagination!)

1 ½ heaping (very packed) cups of cilantro leaves
½ heaping (very packed) cup of parsley
3 garlic cloves, minced
2 small green onions (red onion also works), finely chopped
¼ cup raw red wine vinegar
¼ cup olive oil
¾ teaspoon sea salt or more to taste
¼ teaspoon red pepper flakes (do not use if you can't have anything too spicy; more or less to taste if you are using)

Into food processor, add red wine vinegar and olive oil first. Add the herbs, garlic, and onions a little at a time, blending and scraping down the sides between additions. Once these are all processed add sea salt and red pepper flakes. Taste and add more sea salt as needed.
Transfer to a small bowl or jar.

Thickly slice 6–8 radishes (any variety) to serve on the side.

Now to make the steak...
Individual serving size = ½-1 cup (make an extra cup for lunch tomorrow)
Season the grass-fed skirt steak (can sub flank steak) with salt and pepper and grill over a hot fire until the meat is seared on the outside and rare within, about 2 minutes per side. (Or cook under your broiler the same way; it might take a few minutes more) Transfer to a carving board and let rest for 5 minutes. Thinly slice the steak across the grain. Serve right away, passing the chimichurri sauce at the table.

For tomorrow's lunch...
Shred 1 cup steak for tacos

Chop ½ cup tomato, ¼ cup red onion, ½ cup green or red cabbage, 2 radishes, ½ cup avocado (tips: toss avocado with lemon juice to help prevent blackening and enhances flavor of tacos), ½ cup cilantro. Grab ¼ cup of sprouts and/or microgreens (best if a variety of four kinds together).

Package steak in one container and "toppings" in another and sprouts or microgreens in another. Wrap up a couple of cauliflower tortillas, nori sheets or romaine leaves, depending on what you choose to use as your "tortilla".

Put your wild rice to soak for tomorrow's dinner. (see recipe for instructions)

Day 2
Breakfast:
How to properly cook an egg...
There is much debate these days over whether eggs are healthy or not. Eat just the whites or just the yolks? It can all be rather confusing. Eggs are actually one of nature's almost complete perfect foods. The trick is to cook them slowly at a low temperature so as to preserve the benefits. When cooked at low temperature, slowly, they preserve the healthy cholesterol. When cooked at a higher temp they can produce toxins that adhere to body tissues and cause inflammation.

Perfect Poached Eggs on a bed of sautéed spinach...
This is the best way (but not only way; remember variety applies to cooking methods too) to prepare your eggs because poached eggs are heated gradually and actually become an alkalinizing food when prepared this way, thereby easing the stress on your digestive system.

Bonus tip: To make sure you are using fresh pasture eggs try this trick. Place your egg(s) in a bowl of water. Fresh eggs will sink and lie sideways; older eggs (that are about a week old) will lie on the bottom but bob up and down slightly; three-week-old eggs will balance in the water on their small tips; eggs that float to the surface are bad, and shouldn't be eaten.

Use a wide, shallow pan. Fill the pan about 2/3 with filtered water; this helps you gently place the egg into the water, instead of dropping it in.

Simmer, don't boil. Boiling will break apart the egg white. Add about 1 or 2 teaspoons of apple cider vinegar to the water, which helps the egg white set. Add one egg at a time. Crack the egg into a cup or ramekin first, then gently slide the egg into the water. Cook for about 3 to 5 minutes. The whites should look "set."

While your eggs are finishing up, sauté spinach in butter until wilted. Put spinach in circular rounds on serving plates.

Use a slotted spoon or spatula to lift the egg out of the water and pat the bottom of the spoon dry to remove water before putting the egg on the bed of spinach.

Serve with a side of microgreens and/or sprouts, four different varieties all together to form a medley, and a tablespoon of your favorite sauerkraut. (Top microgreen/sprout medley with some basic dressing if you wish.)

Lunch:

<u>Steak Tacos</u>...Makes 2–4 tacos depending on what kind of "tortilla" you are using

> 1 cup shredded steak (from last night's dinner) (can toss with 1 teaspoon of chimichurri sauce – optional)
>
> ½ cup tomato, chopped
> ¼ cup red onion, chopped
> ½ cup red or green cabbage, chopped
> ½ cup cilantro, chopped
> ½ cup sprouts or microgreens, any blend
> ½ cup avocado, chopped and tossed in lemon juice

Lay out your cauliflower tortilla(s) <u>or</u> romaine <u>or</u> nori sheet(s). Top first with steak, then layer other condiments as you choose on top. Eat immediately with some thickly sliced radishes on the side. For grab n go, take steak in one container, the rest of the ingredients in another, and tortillas or substitutes in another separate container. When lunchtime comes lay out your tortilla or substitute, layer the steak and toppings, and enjoy!

Dinner:

Note: I often double or triple this recipe, soak it on Saturday night, make it on a Sunday cooking it on low for 4 hours in my crockpot so I have extra on hand in the fridge for quick meals. If you are going to make this in the crockpot just add soaked rice, salt and broth to crockpot and cook on low for 4 hours. When it's done add the butter and herbs, mix and it's all set.

Fun Fact: Wild rice when prepared this way counts as a protein

<u>Savory Wild Rice</u>

Serves 2-4
*Night before:
> 1 cup wild rice
> ¼ cup water kefir
> 1 cup filtered water

Combine the wild rice with the water and water kefir, mix well, cover loosely and soak overnight until ready to cook.

For cooking you will need:
> Soaked, drained wild rice
> Bone broth as needed
> 1 tablespoon Herbs de Provence
> 1 teaspoon sea or pink Himalayan salt
> 1 tablespoon grass-fed butter

When ready to cook your rice, strain off any liquid left over. Put your soaked rice in a sauce pot (I love cooking this in a clay pot), cover with whatever bone broth you have up to 1 inch over the top level of the rice. Add herbs de Provence and salt, stirring to mix. Bring to a slow boil on low heat and let simmer until liquid is all absorbed, approximately 30 minutes. Remove from heat, stir to fluff; add 1 tablespoon grass-fed butter and mix well. Serve with a side of microgreens or sprout medley. My favorite combination with this is sunflower sprouts, broccoli, red cabbage, and amaranth microgreens and I top the rice with them as garnish. Rice keeps for up to four days in the fridge and is great warmed up, as you will find out since you are using the remainder for breakfast tomorrow.

While your rice is cooking:

Make the pesto for lunch tomorrow and prepare your wraps for grab 'n' go if needed. Make the balsamic vinaigrette.

Five minutes before your rice is ready, prep your radicchio and place under the broiler. Do not take your eyes off of it as it only takes a second to burn.

Braised Radicchio...
Serves 2

> 1 large or 2 smaller heads of radicchio

Cut the butt end off the radicchio and separate the leaves. (If you choose you can chop the leaves into a fine shred). Arrange the leaves on a cookie sheet and place under your broiler for 2–5 minutes until the leaves are starting to wilt. Do NOT burn! Keep watching it. Remove from the oven and drizzle with balsamic vinaigrette and top with microgreens or sprouts (if you haven't added them to your wild rice) and serve immediately.

Balsamic Vinaigrette...
Makes about 1 cup

> ¾ cup extra-virgin olive oil
> ¼ cup balsamic vinegar
> Sea or pink Himalayan salt
> Fresh-ground black pepper

Optional extras: spoonful of Dijon mustard, minced shallots, minced garlic, minced fresh herbs, teaspoon dried herbs, spoonful of raw honey or coconut sugar.

Combine the olive oil and balsamic in a small jar or other container with a sealed lid. Add a big pinch of salt and a few grinds of black pepper. Screw on the lid and shake vigorously. Dip a piece of lettuce into the vinaigrette and taste. Adjust the salt, pepper, or the proportion of oil and vinegar to taste.

Day 3:

Breakfast:

Wild Rice Hash Bowl

Serves 2

> 2 cups Savory Wild Rice from last night's dinner
> ¼-½ pound ground turkey (or any kind of meat) (optional)
> 2 cups any leftover cooked veggies you have on hand (you should have some peas)
> 2 tablespoons + 1 tablespoon ghee
> 1 tablespoon miso, unpasteurized, any flavor
> 2 tablespoons ginger beet sauerkraut; or you can use any "flavor" and a beet-based one goes great with this recipe
> 4 tablespoons microgreens or sprouts, any combination of at least four varieties
> 2 tablespoons pumpkin seeds, soaked, fermented, sprouted and dehydrated; any nut or seed ready to eat can be subbed here (optional)
> 2 tablespoons sheep feta (optional)
> 1–2 sheets raw nori

Melt 1 tablespoon of ghee in skillet. When melted add ground turkey or other meat if using and cook until browned. Add leftover wild rice and veggies to skillet with 2 tablespoons of ghee. When hot, split this mixture between two bowls. Add ½ tablespoon miso to each bowl and mix well with hot ingredients. Add 1 tablespoon of sauerkraut to each bowl and mix well. Sprinkle with pumpkin seeds (or whatever you're using) and feta (if using). Break up 1 sheet of nori and mix into rice mixture. Top with microgreens and/or sprouts and serve immediately.

Lunch:

Scrumptious Pistachio Pesto Wraps...

Serves 1-2

Note: I often double this recipe so I have extra pesto on hand in the fridge for quick meals or to add to a breakfast wrap or a salad.

> ½ cup shelled, soaked, fermented, sprouted pistachios
>
> 1 teaspoon garlic, minced or pressed
>
> 1 tablespoon unpasteurized miso, any "flavor"
>
> 1 cup fresh basil, lightly packed
>
> 2 teaspoons lemon juice
>
> ¼ cup avocado
>
> 2 tablespoons nutritional yeast
>
> 1 teaspoon dulse flakes
>
> ½ tablespoon pistachio or olive oil (optional)

Add pistachios to your food processor and pulse to chop up a bit. Then add rest of ingredients except basil and oil. Process until almost smooth. Drizzle oil in if using, while pulsing to blend. Add basil and pulse to mix well. Set aside.

Wraps...

> 2 large romaine leaves
>
> 2 sheets raw nori (if using; can just wrap in romaine leaves by themselves)
>
> ¼ cup cucumber, (Persian or lemon my favorites) cut into thin sticks

½ cup microgreens or sprouts, any kinds

Lay romaine leaf down on edge of nori sheet, spread mixture onto leaf and roll. The romaine leaf keeps nori from getting soggy and falling apart. This way it can be made ahead and rolled in parchment paper.

Place about a tablespoon of pesto as a row down the middle of the romaine leaf. Layer cucumber sticks and sprouts and/or microgreens on top. Roll and enjoy! Serve with whatever leftover cooked veggie you have on hand.

Dinner:
Love Those Heirlooms Marinara Sauce...
Serves 2

> 1 ½ cups tomato, chopped (use heirlooms if you can – so worth it!!)
> 1 tablespoon fresh parsley or 1 teaspoon dried
> 2 teaspoons each fresh or 1 teaspoon dried of oregano, thyme
> 6-10 good size fresh basil leaves or 1 teaspoon dried
> ½ teaspoon fresh rosemary or ¼ teaspoon dried
> ½ teaspoon garlic, about 1 small clove, chopped
> 1 tablespoon lemon juice (use Meyer lemons if you can)
> 1 tablespoon pine nuts or walnuts (optional)
> ½ tablespoon nutritional yeast
> ¼ cup of raw, unrefined olive oil (add more if necessary to reach desired consistency)
> ½ teaspoon sea or pink Himalayan salt
> ½ teaspoon fresh ground black pepper (optional)
> 1 tablespoon grated Parmesan or Pecorino Romano, for garnish (optional)

Place all ingredients in high-speed blender and blend until smooth. Set aside to let flavors "blend" while preparing rest of dinner. If you wish, you may gently warm this sauce but do not boil or let it bubble, in order to preserve the nutrients and antioxidants.

Meat option: ground beef, lamb, venison or turkey - brown your meat in medium skillet with garlic, dried thyme, oregano, salt and pepper. If you wish to keep your sauce raw, then pour sauce over the meat with the heat off and let sit covered while you prep your zoodles or noodles. If you wish to warm the sauce slightly more then turn heat to low, pour sauce over meat and gently bring to warm. Turn heat off (and remove if not a gas stove) and cover for 10 minutes.

Kelp noodles: place in bowl and rinse very well. Drain well before using and squeeze out moisture. Toss with olive oil and salt. You can also warm your "noodles" on low heat should you wish but again do not use high heat. After you finish making the salad, come back and layer your noodles with your sauce. Garnish with a sprig of fresh basil and if you wish, dust with some Parmesan or Pecorino cheese, or for a non-dairy option a tad bit more nutritional yeast.

Zoodles: use your spiralizer to turn out beautiful spirals of zucchini. Note: you can sub any vegetable here depending on your tastes. (If you don't have a spiralizer then just cut into thin strips by hand). Toss your zoodles with salt and let sit in a colander to drain for 20 minutes. Then use a towel to press excess moisture out and put in a serving bowl. (if you don't do this, your noodles will be bland and will water down your sauce and detract from the flavor of your sauce.) Optional: toss your zoodles with olive oil first before topping off. You can also warm your zoodles slightly at this point if you wish. Top with marinara or meat sauce and same garnishes, as with the kelp noodles.

Multiple choices:
1. Kelp noodles with marinara sauce
2. Kelp noodles with meat sauce
3. Zoodles with marinara sauce
4. Zoodles with meat sauce

Serve with:

Seasonal salad...
Serves 2

> 3 cups of mesclun mix, or your favorite in-season lettuces
> ½ cup of sprouts and/or microgreens, any kind(s) (I like to mix several kinds for extra flavor and nutrients.)
> 2 tablespoons of your favorite sauerkraut
> ½ cup chopped cucumber, or whatever is in season
> 2 tablespoons soaked, fermented, sprouted seeds or nuts
> 1 large or 2 small purple or red radishes, (if in season) thinly sliced
> 1 tablespoon fresh thyme, oregano and whatever fresh seasonal herbs you love (or any favorite herb combination)
> 1 tablespoon of favorite raw or European cheese (optional)
> 1-2 tablespoons fresh lightly cooked seasonal veggies – (can be cooked and left over from another meal)

Add all ingredients to a large bowl and toss with Rockin' Dressing

Rockin' Dressing...

> ½ cup raw, unrefined olive oil, flax oil or hemp oil. (If you wish to mix oils, use ¼ cup olive oil with ¼ cup hemp or flax oil)

¼ cup apple cider vinegar

¼ cup unpasteurized miso, any "flavor"

1 tablespoon wheat-free, low sodium tamari or nama shoyu (raw soy sauce)

1 tablespoon nutritional yeast

¼ teaspoon spirulina (optional)

¼ teaspoon raw honey (optional)

Pinch of black pepper (optional)

Place all ingredients in blender and blend until smooth. Makes about 1 cup of dressing.

Did you notice how the foods were combined in the meals and throughout the day? Putting together a 5+5 meal really isn't that difficult.

Did you notice that a variety of 4 microgreens/sprouts were in every meal? Curious as to why? Here are some fun facts:

Fun facts:

Sprouts/microgreens

- can contain up to 100 times more enzymes than raw fruits and vegetables, allowing your body to extract more vitamins, minerals, amino acids and essential fats from the foods you eat
- during sprouting, minerals such as calcium and magnesium bind to protein, making them more bioavailable
- are the ultimate locally-grown food, and can easily be grown in your own kitchen, so you know exactly what you're eating, and since they're very inexpensive, cost is no excuse for avoiding them

- sprouts and microgreens do double duty in the 5 + 5 equation; not only are they your 4 raw vegetables, but as they are a micro-protein also cover your 4 raw proteins. Always having several (I aim for at least 4) varieties on hand makes putting together meals which allow your nutrients to be bioavailable a cinch!

Shopping list for 3 Day Sample Menu and Required Make-Ahead Items

(Please note if you are going to double or increase the recipe serving sizes you will need to adjust this shopping list accordingly as well)

It is a given that the ingredients listed below are "organic", pastured, raw and unprocessed. I have listed the minimum amounts for staples such as coconut oil, olive oil, and so on, but go ahead and buy a larger size if you know you will use it again as it will save you money and you might already have many of these items on hand.

Meat

Skirt or flank steak, grass-fed – ¾-1 pound

Ground turkey, pasture raised – ¼-½ pound (if using for Wild Rice Hash)

Ground beef, lamb, grass-fed or venison – ½-¾ pound (if using in Heirloom Marinara Sauce)

Bones, beef, grass-fed (for bone broth)

Liver, beef, grass-fed – 1 medium to large piece (for bone broth)

Fish

1 can wild, line caught sardines, 8 oz or fresh equivalent (if adding to your Red Pepper Soup lunch)

Live Vibrantly! 10 Steps To Maintain Youthfulness, Increase Energy, Restore Your Health

Dairy

Cow, goat, or sheep, raw, hard cheese (I love goat gouda from Europe) – 3 oz (if using cheese)

Parmesan or Pecorino Romano (hard cheese) – 2 oz (if using in Day 1 & 3 dinner)

Feta, —sheep, goat or cow — 5 oz (if using in Wild Rice Hash)

Yogurt — cow, goat or sheep— raw if can get, whole, plain, 6 oz (tip: use as a face mask for fresh, radiant skin!)

Milk, raw – 1 quart goat or cow (for smoothies or other things you use milk for). (If you can't get raw milk I don't recommend any other kind as nothing else has the enzymes and nutrients, which is why it's included in the first place.)

Butter, grass-fed, cow or goat – 8 oz

Pastured eggs – 1 dozen

Fruit

Avocados – 3

Young coconut – 2-3 (if using in breakfasts and you wish to make milk)

Lime – 1

Lemon – 2

Herbs, Fresh

Basil – 1 bunch or package

Oregano – 1 small bunch or package

Thyme – 1 small bunch or package

Rosemary – 1 small bunch or package

Parsley – 1 bunch

Cilantro – 1 large bunch

Dill – 1 small strand (if adding to Red Pepper Soup)

Vegetables

Radicchio – 1 large head or 2 smaller

Microgreens – 4 oz (arugula, broccoli, purple kohlrabi, mizuna, kale; just to name a few)

Sprouts – 4 oz combined (clover, alfalfa, radish, daikon, broccoli, mustard; just to name a few)

Radishes, purple or red – 1 small bunch (slice and add on side of any meal if you have extras; great gallbladder support food)

Tomato, heirloom 4–5

Rocket or arugula – 1 bunch

Romaine – 1 small head

Red bell pepper – 1 medium

Fresh peas (can use frozen) – 1 pound

Green onion – 2 bunches

Spinach – 1 small head or 3 cups baby

Red onion – 1 small

Jalapeno – 1 small (if using)

Cucumber – 1 English or regular or 3 Persian

Seasonal lettuce – 1 head or ½ pound mix

Zucchini – 3 medium

Cauliflower – 1 large head (for tortillas)

Cabbage, red or green – ½ a medium head (if using for tacos)

Nuts/Seeds

Chia seeds – 1-2 cups (if using in cereal and/or smoothie)

Flax seeds (grind yourself best) – ½ cup if using in smoothies

Cashews, raw – 1 cup

Walnuts, raw, shelled – 1 cup

Pine nuts, raw – ¼ cup

Pumpkin seeds, raw – ½ cup

Pistachio, raw, shelled – ½ cup

Almonds, raw – 4 cups (for crackers)

Sea vegetables
Dulse flakes – 2 oz
Nori sheets, raw – 6 sheets, small pack
Kelp noodles – 24 oz

Superfoods
Maca powder – 2 oz
Spirulina – 5 oz
Green powder blend, raw – 4 oz (if using in smoothie)
Nutritional yeast – 8 oz
Raw cacao powder – 6 oz

Spices/Herbs, Dried
Cinnamon – 2 oz
Cardamom, ground – 2 oz (if choosing to use in chia cereal)
Salt, pink Himalayan or sea – small bottle
Black Pepper – 2 oz
Chipotle – 2 oz
Dill – 2 oz
Cumin, ground – 2 oz
Herbs de Provence – 2 oz
Red pepper flakes – 2 oz (if using in Chimichurri sauce)
Paprika – 2 oz (if using in tortillas)
Oregano – 2 oz
Garlic, powder – 2 oz (for crackers)

Oils
Coconut oil – 8 oz
Olive oil – 8 oz

Ghee – 4 oz

Condiments
Coconut butter – 6 oz (can sub coconut oil and save some $)
Miso, unpasteurized – 8 oz
Garlic – 1 large head
Red wine vinegar – 4 oz
Apple cider vinegar, raw, unfiltered – 6 oz
Sauerkraut, raw, unpasteurized – 6 oz (sauerkraut with beets added to it is recommended to go with these recipes but really anything from just basic traditional cabbage to any other "flavor combo" will work)

Miscellaneous
Honey, raw – 6 oz
Wild rice – 4 cups

Tips for Travel and Eating Out

At this point you are probably thinking, "Well, this is all fine and dandy if I never eat out or travel or attend special occasions or events." These situations can be a little tricky and here are some tips to help you navigate them. The key pieces to remember in all of these situations are:

- it's what you do 80% of the time that makes the biggest difference in your life, leaving room for 20% to play with;
- you might not always have the most optimal choices available, and making the best choice for you in that moment in any given situation is most important;
- make your choice, then let it go; don't dwell on it, move on.

For travel:

Live Vibrantly! 10 Steps To Maintain Youthfulness, Increase Energy, Restore Your Health

Before I go somewhere I usually search online in that area for natural food stores and farmers markets, or call the hotel (or friends) where I will be staying and ask them what's around and available. Look for restaurants that serve locally sourced foods and rotate their menus so they are seasonal. Find a local juice bar; there are more and more of these around these days. I also try to take "travel food items" with me as much as I can. What does that look like? For example, when I travel by car I like to bring several staples with me (usually I have a small cooler) such as wild caught canned fish, dried seaweeds/nori sheets, seeds/nuts that have been soaked, fermented, sprouted and dehydrated, spirulina, maca, raw cacao powder, homemade crackers, a block of European hard cheese, homemade nut pate or pesto, grass-fed butter, sauerkraut, sprouts* (hardier than microgreens), coconut oil, fermented vegetable juices, water kefir and/or kombucha, carrots, cucumber, apples, (or other seasonal veggies and fruits that travel well) shaker cup and/or travel blender. With these items I can make quite a combination of meals and supplement with bought items along the way.

*if I'm going to be gone for 5 or more days I actually take my Easy Sprouters (two of them; one for keeping the ready to eat sprouts and the other to sprout a new batch so I don't run out in between) and seeds with me and sprout batches while travelling. I've actually taken my Easy Sprouters out into the backcountry and desert with me while hiking and sprouted as I go for a fresh, live, nutrient-dense food. They are extremely lightweight and so worth having on any trip.

When traveling by plane you run into the dilemma of everything being exposed to radiation. Though these doses are much lower than what they use to irradiate food (which you wish to avoid), that still does not mean your food is not affected. For me it depends on where

I am traveling to. If I know I can get healthy food where I am going, taking my own food is not a huge consideration. If I'm unsure or know my choices will be limited, I will take a few things with me such as canned fish, seaweeds, raw green powder, chia seeds, spirulina, nut/seed blends, coconut oil, and crackers. I can't tell you how many times I have ended up in a situation where there has been nothing I could eat, as I am allergic to wheat and cow dairy, and my travel food has saved me. There are moments when my radiated food might be the best choice of what is available in any moment. My travel blender takes up the same amount of room as a pair of shoes, weighs about the same and comes with a container I can take with me on the go. With my nuts/seeds, raw green powder, coconut oil, chia seeds, spirulina and filtered water, I can always make myself a shake to nourish me. And as already mentioned I love my Easy Sprout and seeds to travel with.

When eating out:

Depending on where you live, eating out might not be the challenge that it is for some. These days many metropolitan areas have restaurants that serve hormone-free meats, organic, traditionally prepared, local and seasonal produce. Even fast food chains are getting on board. You have Chipotle, Carl's Jr., A&W, Sweet Greens, Dig Inn, Elevation Burger, Tender Greens, just to name a few of the bigger chains that now serve hormone-free meat options, and some also serve organic vegetables. Eating at home is your best bet for maintaining your vibrancy and keeping more money in your wallet, and for those special times when you are eating out; have fun. Enjoy your time, the people you are with and the occasion. Smile at your waiter. Ask for suggestions.

A tip I like to recommend is to scan the ingredients in all the offerings. Then I find something that appeals to me the most and meets my requirements and desires in that moment. Sometimes combining appetizers is the way to go. I always skip the bread, potato, pasta (heavy starches) and ask for a double serving of the vegetable. I'm always looking for sprouts of any kind on a menu and will ask to be sure, because you never know. If I have to make substitutions, to keep it simple I ask for ingredients I see on the menu. I'm known for taking my own sprouts/microgreens and wheat-free tamari when I go out to eat. Keep the veggies your largest portion, and supplement with protein. Avoid cream sauces, deep-fried and other such items at places that are not serving grass-fed, pastured or non-GMO products.

Or you can decide it's one of your 20% options, eat whatever and enjoy every mouthful.

At the office:

Take your food to work with you! Again, reserve eating out for special occasions. That doesn't mean you have to stay in the office to eat, though. It's always a good idea to step out if you can on your lunch hour. Take your lunch to an outdoor spot to eat if at all possible. You'll notice how the 3-day menu plan incorporates leftovers from dinner for breakfasts and lunches, in order to keep things simple.

Now before you move into the actual *Live Vibrantly* 10 step blueprint, go to the journaling pages and answer the before you begin questions. These will help you get clear on what you wish to get out of this book and how to use it in your life.

"Wondering how to turn this 10 Step Blueprint into your life? Go to: http://ilivevibrantly.com/programs/live-vibrantly-series/

There you will find the Live Vibrantly! 21 Day Reset To Maintain Youthfulness, Increase Energy, Restore Your Health online program. 21 Days where I walk you through transforming your life step by step. Your vibrant self awaits you. Start your journey now. Go to: http://ilivevibrantly.com/programs/live-vibrantly-series/ to find out how."

Part 3

<u>The Rest of It</u>

Up to this point our primary focus has been on food. And though it plays a huge role in your *Live Vibrantly* 10 step blueprint, there are other factors involved as well. Besides the food you consume, what else is there? Look around you! From the moment you get up in the morning until you lie down at night there are multiple layers that ask to be looked at. Let's start with that scenario.

Lifestyle

You just woke up; you get up and head to the bathroom to start getting ready for your day. If you don't have a whole-house filtration system, do you use filters on your shower? What toothpaste do you use? What skincare? Haircare? Are there chemicals in these? Would you eat it? If not, you shouldn't be using it. Your skin is your largest organ and absorbs everything directly into your bloodstream. Is your toilet paper earth friendly? Look at everything else you have and use in your bathroom and ask these same questions — would you eat it, is it toxic and is it earth friendly.

Now you head into your kitchen and do the same thing, and ask the same questions. Look around, really see what products you use in your kitchen for cleaning, to prepare food, to store food. Are there Teflon products, plastics and other chemical leaching items? What kind of dish soap do you use? Are your paper products earth friendly? Do you have a water filter on your sink if you don't have an entire house filtration system?

I think you're starting to get the idea. This is a noticing exercise, so don't panic about what you notice, don't beret yourself, no guilt allowed. Truly the first step is to notice what you use and what surrounds you in every part of your home. What could you replace with a choice that supports your living vibrantly? The next step is to research what items you would like to replace these with when they need replacing. If you have a health issue you are working with, though, I do recommend switching things out sooner rather than later. Make your list and have it ready for when your items run out. Don't be overwhelmed by your list if it's kind of long. Just pick one thing at a time and eventually you will get through it.

Next, look around you at the space you live in. Does it make you feel good to be in it? Is it clean? Is it moldy? Many don't realize they have a mold issue until it is a serious problem. Check your home frequently to make sure you don't have this issue. Is it cluttered, overflowing with stuff, disorganized, dark? Your space is a reflection of you. If you wish to live vibrantly then your space needs to reflect that as well. If it needs decluttering, don't be overwhelmed. You have options. Look for friends, resources and agencies that will help you sort through things. Or if you wish to do it yourself, do one small thing at a time. Clean off one shelf, for instance. Decide what you absolutely need to keep and what you can re-gift, donate or recycle. Clean that shelf, see it shine. Feel good about your accomplishment; this will keep you motivated. Realize that decluttering is an ongoing beautiful process. Make a commitment to yourself to do a little piece each day, or once a week, until you are caught up.

Look around your bedroom. It should be free of electrical devices such as TV's, smartphones, tablets, electric clocks, phones and electrical devices in support of number 9 of the blueprint. The electromagnetic fields, along with the blue light these emit, interrupt healthy sleep patterns as well as support health imbalances. Eliminating nighttime EMF exposure and blue light is foundational to good health and living vibrantly. EMF's interrupt your body's ability to repair and rejuvenate at a cellular level. They impede melatonin production. They interrupt your natural deep sleep cycles by not allowing the body to go to and stay in a deep sleep.

To recap:
- all personal care and household cleaning items should be nontoxic and environmentally friendly
- all cooking apparatus and utensils should be nontoxic and safe

- filtration devices should be used for household drinking and bathing water at the very least
- your bedroom should be free of electrical devices, especially cell/smartphones (even if they are turned off), TV's, and cordless phones

More lifestyle tips to support you to *Live Vibrantly*:

- Take 3-5 deep breaths before beginning to eat any food; that turns your digestion "on." (This tip works into number 8 of the blueprint.)

  Okay, simple enough, 3-5 deep breaths before you eat. Why is this important, though? Most people think they open their mouth, insert food and magically digestion happens, yes? NO! It doesn't just happen.

  Our bodies function in two different modes, sympathetic or parasympathetic. Sympathetic nervous system is the fight or flight mode, the one that most individuals are in most of the time due to stress, busy work and life schedules. Parasympathetic is the calm, relaxed mode of the nervous system.

  Many people shovel food into their mouths while working, driving, watching TV or doing some other activity. This keeps them in sympathetic mode where that switch is on. If the "switch" is not flipped off then parasympathetic mode doesn't happen, which means digestion will not happen.

When digestion is not allowed to happen then digestive problems arise. The nutrients from your food will not get to your cells, leading to deficiencies. Your gut communicates with your brain all the time so not only does your mood affect how you digest, but when you do not digest properly your mood is altered.

You can support your digestive system and prevent issues by stopping to take 3-5 deep breaths before you start putting food in your mouth, which will turn off the sympathetic mode and put you into parasympathetic mode.

This practice usually helps you to slow down and chew your food as well. Worried you only have 10 minutes to eat your lunch? Try this — stop whatever you are doing, take 5 deep breaths, take smaller mouthfuls and chew your food well. Focus on nothing else for those 10 minutes. I promise, even if you don't finish your portion, you will feel more satisfied, brighter and more energized from what you did get to eat than if you had raced to shovel it all in and finish the portion. Remember, breath is your life force and plays a very important part in nourishing your body. Breathe, deeply. Not just before you eat but throughout the day.

- Sauna once a week or at least twice a month for at least 20 minutes up to 40 minutes. Rinse off with Dr. Bronners (or some kind of castile soap) and cold water afterwards, and/or take a 20 minute bath once a week with Epsom salts or your favorite bath salts and essential oils. Rinse with cold or cooler water afterwards. This supports detoxification and reduces the toxic load on the body.

I know some of you go to great lengths to avoid sweating but it really is good for you! Not only does it cool you down but it rids the body of waste products. Sweating mobilizes toxins stored in the fat and enhances their elimination. Every day you are exposed to pollutants and environmental toxins. Taking a sauna or a detox bath helps to counteract and release these from your body. It's also good for your heart; like mild exercise. The heart gets a gentle workout while the heat of the sauna dilates the capillaries and improves blood flow.

The body contains two main types of sweat glands:

- **Apocrine glands**, located mostly in the armpits, pubic area and scalp, secrete sweat that contains fats and other organic compounds. (Bacteria on the skin interacting with these compounds is what causes body odor.) These glands, which become functional at puberty, also emit hormones and pheromones believed to attract the opposite sex.

- **Eccrine glands**, which number more than 2 million and are scattered all over the body, are the real workhorses when it comes to sweating. Activated by heat as well as stress and emotions, these glands secrete odorless, watery sweat that cools you down as it evaporates on the skin.

I prefer far-infrared saunas as they are easier to fit into your home, less expensive, easy to install, do not require plumbing and use minimal amounts of energy. Because they do not heat the air, you can usually stay in one of these longer than a regular sauna. Personally, I aim for the bath once a week and sauna once a week. You will really notice the difference in how you feel when you practice both or at least one of these.

- Expose yourself to 10–20 minutes of natural outdoor light daily, without sunscreen:

This is number 7 of the blueprint. I can just hear you exclaiming over the no sunscreen part! And yes, you got it right, outside, in the sun with no sunscreen! Why on earth would I suggest this?

Let's break it down. There are 17 FDA-approved chemicals that go into sunscreen. Fifteen of those are clear chemicals that absorb UV light and 2 are minerals that reflect UV light. Of these 15, nine are known endocrine disruptors. That means that they interfere with the normal function of hormones. Whoa, endocrine disruptors, seriously??!! And skin is your largest organ; anything you put on it goes directly to your blood stream. These 15 chemicals don't just sit on the surface of your skin, they scatter all over the body without being detoxified by the liver and can be detected in blood, urine, and breast milk for up to two days after a single application. Do you want those nine chemicals wandering around in your body causing problems?

So what about natural sunscreens? Read the labels. Most of these have chemicals in them that you wouldn't eat so why put them on your skin for your body to "eat?" If you do find one that is completely made from ingredients that won't harm you then it is good to have on hand for those times when you will be in full sun for an extended time or out on the water all day.

Heliotherapy is the term for sun as therapy and goes way back. Think about it! Plants and animals need the sun to survive and thrive, why should we be any different? Heliotherapy has been used in the following situations successfully:
- Acne, psoriasis and other skin disorders
- Muscular stimulation and relaxation
- Seasonal Affective Disorder
- Reducing body odor
- Boosting the body's immune system for the treatment of AIDS
- Reducing bacteria count from infections by as much as 50%.

Another reason you don't want sunscreen for these quick exposures is so that your body absorbs the light that helps us make Vitamin D from the sun. The best times to get this light are between 10am and 2pm, but really just getting outside in the daylight anytime is good for you. Another surprising factor about eating according to the blueprint is you should not burn as easily as you have in the past.

Vitamin D protects us from many health issues and is deficient in most people these days. Dr. Mercola calls vitamin D "one of the simplest solutions to wide-ranging health problems." It helps keep hormones balanced and fight infection from the bad bacteria and viruses. I also recommend a good whole food vitamin supplement foundation program to my clients that includes vitamin D with K.

- Walk 1-3 times a week outdoors in nature for a minimum of 30 minutes. Keeping the   body moving prevents stagnation and supports the body to de-stress:

Just as you have a "stress" button, you also have a "relaxation" button. Nothing triggers that better than taking a walk in nature. Of course, walking in general will help reduce stress hormones by clearing your head and boosting endorphins but walking outside in nature can actually put your body into a state of meditation. Really! Psychology calls it "involuntary attention" which means something holds our attention while simultaneously allowing for reflection. Walking in green space also helps conquer mental fatigue and even boost cognitive functioning.

- Drink filtered water; wash all your food in it and cook with it for protection from parasites and toxic chemicals. This is in support to number 4 of the blueprint. Install shower and tap filters to remove chlorine (which becomes toxic gas in the shower) and fluorine so skin and food do not absorb them and take them into the body; reduce toxic chemical and heavy metal load on body. Is it really that important to use a filtration system? What is in tap water?

It's chlorinated. It's fluoridated. It's contaminated with pharmaceuticals and other chemicals. Yes, you've heard it a thousand times but have you really stopped to ponder what that means? All of these destroy the good bacteria in your gut and body causing huge imbalances in your microbiome. Fluoride is a poison with no benefit to humans whatsoever. A New York Times article said:

"Only 91 contaminants are regulated by the Safe Drinking Water Act, yet more than 60,000 chemicals are used within the United States, according to Environmental Protection Agency estimates. Government and independent scientists have scrutinized thousands of those chemicals in recent decades, and identified hundreds associated with a risk of cancer and other diseases at small concentrations in drinking water," according to an analysis of government records by The New York Times. Many of these chemicals have not been tested since the 70's or 80's nor has the Safe Drinking Water Act been updated to include many of these, so individuals have been exposed to thousands of toxic and poisonous chemicals over many years without any laws being broken. Filtration devices are worth the investment and impact the health of you and your children greatly for the better. Look for proven ones that remove viruses, parasites and heavy metals.

For the same reason you get a filter for your drinking water you would for your shower.

- Use non-fluoride, sodium lauryl or laureth-free toothpaste; toothpastes without sodium bicarbonate, alcohol sugars and antibacterial ingredients in it. The one I recommend is Revitin; available online at revitin.com in the fall of 2015. Simply put, the chemicals and dyes in commercial toothpastes and oral care products expose you to poisonous chemicals and disrupt your oral microbiome. Most "natural" toothpastes also contain harmful chemicals and antibacterial ingredients that disrupt your oral microbiome and harm your gums and teeth. Diet plays the largest role in your gum and tooth health but your choice of oral care products plays a large role as well. Make a choice that will support your oral microbiome rather than destroy it.

- Keep green plants in each room to improve air quality. Did you know NASA has created a list of the best house plants to improve air quality in your home? Yup. Not only do plants produce oxygen they can also absorb contaminants like benzene and formaldehyde (a known carcinogen). Research also shows that plant-filtered rooms have 50 to 60 per cent less airborne microbes, like mold spores and bacteria. And here is that list:
  Spider plants
  Peace lilies
  Snake plants (aka mother-in-law's tongue)
  Elephant ears
  Weeping figs
  Rubber plants
  Bamboo palms (aka reed palm)

- Walk with bare feet on natural ground/earth 2 times per week for five to ten minutes to dispel stored electrical current; much as ground wire carries away excessive electrical current (called Earthing) (helps reduce EMFs in body). Back in the day, we humans had much more direct contact with the earth. Our skin touched the ground on many occasions. Today not so much; modern life as we know it has us very far removed from these habits. And today we are surrounded by so many currents that interrupt our own electrical field within our bodies and throw it askew. Earthing is your best defense and way to rebalance yourself. And it's so easy and free! Stick bare feet directly on earth, sand, grass, whatever, for five to ten minutes. It doesn't get much easier than that. Yet the benefits can be profound.

- Avoid microwaves and microwaved foods. Microwave cooking robs food of nutrients. Undercooked or unevenly cooked food does not kill parasites.
  Hans Hertel is the first scientist to conceive of and conduct a quality study on the effects of microwaved nutrients on the blood and physiology of human beings. This small but well-controlled study pointed out the degenerative force of microwave ovens and the food produced in them. The conclusion clearly indicated that microwave cooking changed the nutrients so that changes took place in the participants' blood; these were not healthy changes but were changes that could cause deterioration in the human systems. Studies since then have shown that lymphocytes (white blood cells) showed a more distinct short-term decrease following the intake of microwaved food than

after the intake of food cooked by other means. Each of these indicators points the body in a direction away from vibrant health and toward degeneration. The bottom line with microwaves is they alter the molecules in food, taking them from life supporting to life degenerating. Remember life = life; microwaves take the life out of your food.

- Purchase a mini-rebounder and use it for 5-15 minutes a day, 3-5 times a week. You can use this in support of number 6 of the blueprint. It helps move congestion and stagnation in the lymph system; it's a great workout! Your lymph system is the only system in your body to not have its own movement system. It needs your help. Rebounding is one of the best methods to do this. It not only supports your lymphatic system to move and prevent stagnation (read cellulite here as well), it provides many other benefits, some of which are:

  Boosts immune function

  Great for skeletal system and increasing bone mass

  Helps improve digestion

  More than twice as effective as running without the extra stress on the ankles and knees

  Increases endurance on a cellular level by stimulating mitochondrial production (these are responsible for cell energy)

  Helps improve balance by stimulating the vestibule in the middle ear

  Rebounding helps circulate oxygen throughout the body to increase energy.

  Rebounding is a whole body exercise that improves muscle tone throughout the body.

Some sources claim that the unique motion of rebounding can also help support the thyroid and adrenals

- Get plenty of deep, restful sleep. This is number 9 of the blueprint. For some that means 7 hours, for others that could be 9 hours. t. Whatever your needs are, meet them! Interrupted sleep is one of the biggest contributing factors to adrenal, thyroid, hormone and immune issues. It affects every aspect of health and robs you of it. I get that there are circumstances and situations that are beyond your control and know that sometimes it's just not going to happen. But do your best to make it happen. Keep in mind too that a healthy and balanced microbiome supports calm, relaxed, deep, sleep.

- Have fun! Surround yourself with things and people that add to your positive and peaceful well-being; laugh with yourself and friends; forgive yourself and others.

- Take time to notice the beauty in what surrounds you; life is precious, take time to notice and enjoy the moments.

How To Transition Into The *Live Vibrantly* Lifestyle

Living vibrantly is a lifelong journey; it doesn't end until you are no more. Change doesn't just happen overnight. The whole process is about doing the best you can every day, moment by moment. Notice how certain choices make you feel, be aware of how your environment affects you. Make changes that contribute to you and your family feeling great. There is no deprivation involved here. Expand your horizons and open the door to new things. Many get stuck in a rut of eating the same foods cooked and prepared the same way over and over, doing the same workouts all the time, walking the same routes. Change things up! Yes, you may have your favorites and that's great, but what else is out there? Challenge yourself; find out!

Include the whole family. When you have a family and everyone's favorite foods or activities are different this can be more of a challenge. Involve everyone in the process, though. Explain why changes are being made and how important they are. Go to the farmers market as a family. Have kids each plant their own flower, herb or vegetable and be responsible for its care and harvest. Decide on and create recipes as a group; cook together at least one meal a week. Have each person pick an activity each week that the whole family will participate in. Make it fun! Often when kids are involved in the process they take much more of an interest in and offer up less resistance to change. This is a great way to spend more time together as a family, educate yourself and your children, and invest in your children's vibrant future.

So where to start?
Start with your food and meals. Start with one meal a day. I recommend breakfast as it is the most important meal of the day, but

whatever works for you. When you feel comfortable and no longer have to put too much brain effort into pulling off that meal, then move onto the next meal and so on until you have all three main meals down. Along the way you can add special treats and staple items as you can. As you run out of pantry items, restock with better choices if it is needed. As your taste buds get used to fresh, live food and your body starts to feel the difference, previous, perhaps less healthy, choices will naturally phase out. Make large batches of food when you are preparing things so you have options to choose from and spend less time in the kitchen. The goal is to have bits of things already ready to eat in your fridge so you can just choose items and mix and match into different meals and combos, maybe adding a dish every couple of days as you go. Rid your kitchen and pantry of food that does not support living vibrantly. Gather recipes; use your notebook to note what ones are keepers what changes you made to it to make it a 5+5 combo, future suggestions and so on.

Notice. Throughout this book, you have been asked to notice things — how you feel after eating a certain food or meal, how your living environment makes you feel, how you smell and so on. Noticing is one of the biggest steps towards living vibrantly. As you begin to notice what contributes to your vibrancy you will lean more towards those things and those changes. How do you feel when you wake in the morning? Refreshed, alive, ready to leap into your day? How do you feel throughout the day? What contributes to your not feeling good? Once you start to feel great all the time it's harder to make choices that make you feel anything less. Use the observation questions in the journaling section to deepen your awareness around each new habit or piece you incorporate into your life.

Add in lifestyle pieces. Once you start getting the hang of your food and meals, then start looking at the lifestyle pieces and start with one thing at a time. Don't overwhelm yourself or guilt yourself. Pick one place to start. Check that off your list, then move on to the next. It's a process, remember, not an overnight overhaul.

Tips to Make Your Transition:

Baby Steps. Each day or week or month, whatever works for you, choose one small thing you would like to change. Focus your attention on that until you have achieved your goal. Then move on to the next thing. Don't worry about not getting it "perfect" or think you are taking too long. However long it takes you is perfect; it's your timing, it's your life.

Breathe. It's amazing that many people don't realize they go through most of the day holding their breath or only taking quick shallow breaths. It's important to actually take big, long deep belly breaths to keep oxygen flowing through you and especially to your brain. This also switches you out of "stress" mode and into "relaxed" mode. Remember when we talked about that regarding digestion?

Be Grateful. You are going to have less than perfect days; that is life. If you keep waiting for the perfect ideal timing or situation you might spend the rest of your life waiting. Life happens, so make your choices in the moment and be grateful for whatever you choose. Don't add stress or guilt to yourself; that defeats your purpose and goals.

Variety and moderation. These are the most important pieces to remember and live by. Even something good can become harmful when eaten or used to extreme. This applies to food, lifestyle choices, movement, everything.

Other factors that influence how vibrantly you live are how much movement your body gets each day, what you think, and where your thoughts are focused throughout the day.

Movement

You'll notice that I use the term movement as opposed to exercise. It is important to move functionally, move fast and move often. If you've ever watched young children you will notice that though they don't exercise per se, they are always moving. They don't go to gyms or run endless miles but they sprint, climb, race, squat and do many other functional movements constantly. We can take a lesson from that. Think about how you move through your day; how long do you sit without moving? Science has proven that sitting at a desk for extended periods is extremely bad for us. These days there are standing desks, balance boards and walking treadmills. If you have to sit, have you tried sitting on a balance ball? This engages your core, strengthening it as you balance on the ball.

Let's go back to that analogy of the body of water. It is common knowledge that a pool of water with no movement becomes stagnant, building up harmful bacteria, becoming murky, sometimes smelly, and the things in it slowly decompose, whereas a pool of water that has movement stays fresh, clear, bright, maintains its healthy bacteria, smells good, and gives life. Which would you rather be? Your goal should be to move steadily for 20–30 minutes daily, and breaking a sweat makes it even better. This might even look like you putting on your favorite music and dancing as if no one were watching you. Or do this with your kids. Engage them, have fun together. Go for a family walk. The possibilities are endless.

I know you are pretty aware of the benefits of movement on a daily basis and I'll reiterate some fundamental ones here as a reminder.

- Combats illness and dis-ease. Movement boosts HDL, the kind of cholesterol you want, and helps decrease LDL. It helps to keep blood sugar regulated. It can help you prevent or improve metabolic syndrome, type 2 diabetes, depression, certain types of cancer, and arthritis, just to name a few.

- Increases energy. By increasing oxygen, blood flow and nutrients to your tissues and brain it improves your endurance and supports your cardiovascular system to work more efficiently. It also improves muscle strength. When your brain, tissues, lungs and heart are working more efficiently then you work more efficiently.

- Improves your mood. Physical activity stimulates various brain chemicals and hormones that can leave you feeling happier and more relaxed. It also supports your friendly bacteria to stay happy and strong. You may also feel stronger and more aligned with your body when you move regularly, which can boost your appreciation, confidence and love for yourself and what you are capable of doing.

- Helps control toxic buildup in fat cells. When you move on a regular basis, it keeps everything in your body moving and helps prevent toxins from building up and becoming stuck in stagnant areas of your body, especially in fat cells. Remember the pool of water?

- Supports better and deeper sleep. Just don't do too much strenuous movement right before bed. Exception — stretching and relaxing yoga can be beneficial right before bed.

- Puts the spark back into your sex life. Regular physical movement can lead to enhanced arousal for women. And men who engage in consistent movement are less likely to have problems with erectile dysfunction than are men who tend to be sedentary.

Live Vibrantly! 10 Steps To Maintain Youthfulness, Increase Energy, Restore Your Health

<u>Tips and tricks:</u>

Take the stairs whenever you have a choice, park further away in the outskirts of the parking lot, walk or ride a bike instead of driving to the corner store, squat when you have to pick something up. You get the idea. These are among my favorite forms of "movement" besides going for long hikes in nature, yoga and Zumba.

Only attempt this if you are already used to high intensity exercise on a regular basis: Do a fast-paced walk for 5 minutes, then sprint (or other high-intensity exercise) for 20 seconds, recover for 10 seconds (keep walking or moving but slowly so as to rest), keep repeating for a total of three to eight times in 4 minutes. Now rest for 10 seconds. Cool down and stretch for 2 minutes. Quick and effective! Try using these intervals while jumping rope.

It's called <u>The Tabata Protocol</u>. Check out the website for more details, how to get started and background. This is a great fat-burning technique! Even when I have the time for a longer walk I incorporate this protocol into it too.

Note 1: If you are sprinting and not using some sort of machine, do this on real ground, NOT pavement, for best results. Practice this every two days alternated with a 20-40 minute walk. Try to be outside as much as you can.

Note 2: If you have structural issues, injuries or intuitively know your body is not physically ready for this step, then just walk (be sure to swing your arms!) starting for 10-20 minutes and build up to 30, then 40 minutes. Realize that fear is not an excuse; it is your fuel! Challenge yourself!

Your Mind Chatter Matters

YOU are whole. YOU are loved. YOU are valuable. YOU are special. YOU are not alone.

Do you feel the truth of these words resonate in you, deep down in your core?
Or are they just words that float right over you and don't resonate with you at all?

These days there is more and more evidence to support what holistic practitioners have been saying forever, that what you think affects how your body feels. How you "talk" to yourself plays an important role in how your body respond to all the things you do. Improving your food choices, making better lifestyle choices and moving on a regular basis are all important and beneficial, but if you continue to speak to yourself in a negative way then all those beneficial choices can be sabotaged. Negative mind chatter feeds your unfriendly bacteria, not the friendlies, and keeps you from thriving. Positive wellbeing actually plays a larger role in supporting regeneration in your body than food and movement — it's that important! Don't neglect this aspect; you can't thrive without working in this area too.

Positive thinking doesn't mean you are unrealistic and have your head buried in the sand, so to speak. What it does mean is that you recognize you have a choice of how you will respond to any given situation. It doesn't mean you don't feel your emotions. It means you feel them, allow them to move through you, then OUT of you. You don't hold onto them or stay stuck in them. Young children are great examples of this. They feel their emotions fully in the moment, then move through them and onto something else.

Live Vibrantly! 10 Steps To Maintain Youthfulness, Increase Energy, Restore Your Health

Notice how and what you say to yourself makes you feel, on every level. Notice what others say and how they say it makes you feel on every level. Practice speaking to yourself and others in a way that supports you and them to feel loved, whole, and valuable. Often it's not what we say, but how we say it that makes the impact even with ourselves. Do your words inspire you? Inspire others?

I chose the name *I Live Vibrantly* for my practice because it is a positive affirmation statement. Positive affirmations, mantras, and meditations all play a crucial and beneficial role in upping your vibrancy levels. Find and choose what works for you. Experiment, play. Use a combination of things.

One of my favorite exercises that I use with myself and clients is this: Before going to bed, take five minutes; sit comfortably and in stillness in a dark or softly lit space. Make sure you are warm and comfortable. Close your eyes. Breathe slowly and deeply. Starting at your head, scan your body, notice how every part of you feels from head to toe. Give the tense, sore parts permission to relax and feel better. For example, you feel tenseness in your neck and shoulders. You might say something like, "Hello dear neck and shoulders. I acknowledge you are carrying the brunt of my tiredness and stress and will support you in releasing and relaxing. May you be released and rejuvenated through deep sleep tonight." Visualize your neck muscles and shoulder muscles unwinding and releasing their tension while you sleep when you speak your words. Breathe into that space, deeply. Visualize you, your whole body, inside and outside, strong, relaxed, vibrant. Visualize your friendly bacteria doing their job and supporting you to be healthy and happy. Acknowledge one thing you are grateful for from your day. Let go of the day, forgive yourself and anyone else.

At first this may take more than five minutes until you get used to it. If it is taking longer, then either take the extra time or each night focus on a different part of your body. You can do this in the morning or any other time of day if that feels better for you. You can do this more than once a day if you wish. You can do it with your children by asking them questions about how parts of their body feel and teach them the habit of noticing.

I would like to leave you with one of my favorite quotes by Diane Ackerman: "I don't want to get to the end of my life and find that I lived just the length of it. I want to have lived the width of it as well."

May you experience all the health, joy and love you could possibly endure,
~johanna

Now go forth with your newly found knowledge, inspiration, and tools and be the vibrant living soul that is you — live your birthright.

For more information on how you can go deeper into what your body needs, and to find out more about private one on one coaching with me, go HERE. I look forward to supporting you and your uniqueness in your deeper quest to flourish.

Now before you move into the actual *Live Vibrantly* 10 step blueprint, go to the journaling pages and answer the before you begin questions. These will help you get clear on what you wish to get out of this book and how to use it in your life.

"Wondering how to turn this 10 Step Blueprint into your life? Go to: http://ilivevibrantly.com/programs/live-vibrantly-series/
There you will find the Live Vibrantly! 21 Day Reset To Maintain Youthfulness, Increase Energy, Restore Your Health online program. 21

Days where I walk you through transforming your life step by step. Your vibrant self awaits you. Start your journey now. Go to: http://ilivevibrantly.com/programs/live-vibrantly-series/ to find out how."

The Next Stage

Journaling Pages

Before you begin:

1. What motivated me to read this book?

2. Why am I interested in the Live Vibrantly 10 step blueprint?

3. If I lived my life from a place of freedom to be vibrant instead of fear of my body giving out; how would I be different? How would my life be different?

4. What specific symptoms/issues am I hoping to resolve?

5. What do I perceive my challenges to be?

6. I will allow myself to change and become more in harmony with my body because...

7. I will succeed in my journey of living vibrantly because...

Live Vibrantly! 10 Steps To Maintain Youthfulness, Increase Energy, Restore Your Health

As you incorporate each new habit work with these observation questions:

1. What were your challenges trying to incorporate this habit?

2. How did you feel when you did it?

3. How did you feel when you did NOT do it?

4. What did you notice about yourself?

5. What changed for you when you did this daily?

Resources

Proteins List

Fish & Seafood – use the Seafood Watch app on your phone or device, online – seafoodwatch.org

Chicken – pasture raised, bone-in, dark meat preferable, all parts and offal. Use bones/carcass, offal and feet for bone broth.

Turkey – pasture raised, all parts for eating and broth.

Eggs – chicken or duck, truly pasture raised; not fed any grain feed; from local farms are best (yolk may be eaten raw, not whites).

Beef – grass-fed, pasture raised. Use the liver and bones to make a bone broth specifically for healing the microbiome that is rich in collagen (helps reduce and prevent wrinkles and cellulite) amino acids and minerals.

Lamb – grass-fed, pasture raised. Use the liver specifically for thyroid support; it's high in omegas, B vitamins and selenium. Use all parts for eating and for bone broth.

Bison/Buffalo – grass-fed, pasture raised. Use the liver, which is high in protein, omega 3's. Use all parts for eating and bone broth.

Venison and other game meats, whatever you can find or come across, are also great options and support increasing the variety of what you eat. Always try to get or include the offal if you can, especially the liver! Again use all parts for eating and broth.

Live Vibrantly! 10 Steps To Maintain Youthfulness, Increase Energy, Restore Your Health

Sea Vegetables (microprotein and minerals): Nori (sheets that sushi is rolled in), dulse, kombu, sea palm, hijiki, wakame, just to name a few.

Other microproteins/minerals – spirulina, blue green algae, chlorella, wheatgrass, barley grass, oat grass, sprouts and microgreens, (these do double duty as microprotein and raw vegetables), beet greens; wild rice soaked, fermented and cooked slowly at low temperature, legumes soaked, fermented, sprouted and cooked slowly at low temperature.

Proteins: (raw)
Hemp seeds
Flax seeds
Chia seeds
Sesame seeds; black and white*
Almonds*
Cashews*
Pine nuts*
Pumpkin seeds*
Sunflower seeds*
Hazelnuts*
Walnuts*
Pecans*
Brazil nuts*
Macadamias*
Young coconut pulp
Coconut, dried unsweetened
Raw goat milk
Raw cow milk
Cow, goat or sheep cheeses (raw, grass-fed preferably, or European; US rennets and microbials are mostly GMO)

Cow, goat or sheep yogurt – whole, plain (raw, grass-fed preferably)
Whey – cow or goat

*Soak for at least 8 hours, overnight best, using 1 cup of nut or seed with ¼ cup water kefir and 3-4 cups filtered water, rinse, then put on cookie sheet damp and leave to sprout for up to 8 hours, then, if you do not have a dehydrator, place in your oven at 180 degrees to dehydrate until they reach desired crispness.

Note: You can make "pesto" or "nut/seed pates" from nuts or seeds to use as toppings and condiments. Use nutritional yeast instead of cheese if desired, and mix with cilantro, parsley, mint, basil – experiment, have fun!

Live Vibrantly Shopping Template:

This is a template guide for you to use when shopping. Remember what's available varies by season and where you are located. There are spaces at the end of each category for you to add your own items to your list.

Nuts and Seeds:

- almonds (preferably not from California which are all flashpasteurized)

- hazelnuts

- cashews

- pumpkin

- sunflower

- sesame seeds; both black and tan

- walnuts

- pecans

- pistachios

- pine nuts

- brazil nuts

- chia seeds

- hemp seeds

- flax seeds

Dried herbs and spices:

- thyme

- oregano

- basil

- rosemary

- herbs de Provence blend

- cumin

- ground ginger

- turmeric

- curry

- cinnamon

- ground sage

- red pepper flakes

- chipotle powder

- Cajun spice

- sea and pink Himalayan salt

- black pepper

- garlic powder

Oils:

- lard or tallow, from grass-fed animals

- raw extra virgin coconut

- ghee, grass-fed

- avocado oil

- unfiltered extra virgin olive

- flax or hemp

- sesame

- toasted sesame

Vinegars:

•unfiltered raw apple cider

•coconut

•balsamic

•rice

•red wine

Superfoods:

- raw green powder blend containing e3live and blue green algae

- spirulina

- maca powder

- matcha tea or powder

- raw cacao nibs and powder

- raw nori sheets

- wakame

- dulse flakes and strips

- goji berries

- mulberries

Miscellaneous:

- wild, line-caught sardines

- wild, line-caught anchovies

- oysters

- caviar

- capers

- unsweetened shredded coconut

- backup jar of unpasteurized raw miso

- nutritional yeast

- wheat-free tamari or raw shoyu

- raw coconut aminos

- raw, sprouted tahini butter

- raw, sprouted nut butters

- coconut flour

- dates

- vermouth (great with seafood!)

- Madeira (fabulous to cook mushrooms in)

- Chinese rice wine

Sweeteners:

- raw honey

- pure maple syrup

- coconut sugar

Teas:

- raw green powder blend containing e3live and blue green algae

Ancient Grain flours, plus:

- Note: I currently do not have a grain mill so I buy already sprouted flours and usually soak and ferment them before using for breads, muffins, or pancakes.

- organic Einkorn (can be pricey but so worth it, my favorite form of heirloom wheat; low gluten)

- sprouted spelt (next favorite heirloom wheat, not as pricey as Einkorn, also lower gluten)

- sprouted Kamut (another heirloom wheat, less pricey and low gluten)

- sprouted rye

- sprouted blue corn (gluten free)

- sprouted buckwheat (gluten free)

- sprouted amaranth (gluten free)

Fridge and Fresh Produce...

Dairy:

- pastured chicken and/or duck eggs (not actual dairy but usually

  found in that section)

- grass-fed butter, cow or goat

- hard and soft goat or sheep cheese from Europe (not local because

  most of the microbes used in the USA are GMO)

- raw goat milk (or raw cow milk from A2 producing cows also good)

  (to use in smoothies and to make raw homemade yogurt –

  unhomogenized milk next best choice),

- plain yogurt, raw preferably, cow, goat or sheep (I make my own

  using raw goat milk)

Vegetables: (buy according to the season and what's locally available)

- jalapenos

- cucumber – English, Persian, lemon, apple; use a variety of what's in season

- celery

- red and green cabbage (I just have a little piece cut off the head at the store and then stored in a sealed container; it lasts for several weeks in fridge)

- salad greens

- fresh basil

- oregano

- thyme

- parsley

- cilantro

- sprouts and microgreens– several different kinds

- tomatoes

Vegetables: (continue)

- carrots

- red bell pepper

- Poblano or Anaheim peppers

- mushrooms

- whatever else is currently in season

Fruit:

•apples

•lemons (I prefer Meyer)

•limes

•avocados

•young coconuts (not really fruit, but usually stocked in fruit area of

store)

Condiments:

•onion

•garlic

•ginger

•shallots

Meat:

- grass-fed beef or pasture chicken bones for bone broth (or any kind of bones you can get)

- chicken or beef livers (or any kind of offal you can get)

- chicken feet (I always have homemade stock/broth on hand)

- pastured grass-fed beef

- pastured grass-fed bison

- pastured grass-fed lamb or mutton

- venison

- rabbit

- pastured goat

- pastured chicken

- pastured turkey

- pastured duck

- (Look for meats outside of what you normally eat and give them at try; you don't know if you'll like it till you try it! And these are great ways to spread out your budget and get a variety of nutrients. At least once a month try something new.)

Fish and Seafood:

- Fish – use the Seafood Watch app on your phone or device or online for choices – seafoodwatch.org

- Seafood – use the Seafood Watch app on your phone or device or online for choices – seafoodwatch.org

- A good rule of thumb is to stay away from farmed fish and seafood to avoid antibiotics . Also these do not have the nutrients you expect and are looking for.

<u>Foundational recipes:</u>

Basic Dressing...

> 1 level tablespoon unpasteurized miso, any "flavor"
>
> 1 heaping tablespoon tahini, raw, sprouted
>
> 1/2 level tablespoon nama shoyu or wheat-free tamari
>
> 1/4 cup raw apple cider vinegar
>
> 1/2 – 3/4 cups high quality unrefined olive oil (depending on taste)

Add all ingredients to a 16 oz wide-mouth jar with a lid and whisk until creamy, then shake well. Store in fridge between uses. This gets a little solid in the fridge so be sure to take it out first before you begin cooking or assembling food or sit it in a dish of hot water to warm. Goes with just about any type of salad or veggies both raw and cooked.

This dressing is very strong tasting on its own. Paired with salads and veggies it's delightful.

Cauliflower Tortillas...

Makes 6

> 1 head of cauliflower, cut up and stems removed
>
> 2 large eggs
>
> ½ tsp. dried oregano
>
> ½ tsp. paprika
>
> ½ teaspoon of fresh lime juice
>
> Sea salt and freshly ground black pepper

Preheat oven to 375 F.

Using a blender or a food processor, pulse the cauliflower until you get a texture that is finer than rice.

Steam the riced cauliflower over boiling water for 5 minutes.

Place the steamed cauliflower in a dish towel, let it cool for a few minutes (so you don't burn yourself) then squeeze out as much excess water as you can. You should be able to get out a lot of water by being really aggressive about squeezing it. If not, you'll end up with soggy tortillas later.

Transfer the cauliflower to a bowl. Add the eggs, oregano, paprika, lime and seasoning to taste (you can use any spices you like).

Separate the mixture into 6 balls of equal size, and flatten each ball out on a parchment-lined baking sheet to make six small circles.

Place in the oven and bake for 8 to 10 minutes; then flip and cook for another 5 minutes.

Reheat in a pan placed over low heat when ready to serve.

Herbed Almond Crackers...

> 4 cups almond meal (add 3 ½ - 3 ¾ cups of soaked, fermented, sprouted, dehydrated almonds to food processor and grind briefly to get powder meal; do not overgrind or it will turn into nut butter)
> 1 ½ teaspoon sea or pink Himalayan salt
> 1 teaspoon garlic powder or ½ teaspoon fresh garlic, pressed
> 1 teaspoon fresh herb or ½ teaspoon dried (rosemary, basil, herbs de Provence, or Cajun spice all work great; use your imagination, create your own combinations)
> 2 large eggs
> 2 tablespoons melted butter or coconut oil

Preheat oven to 350 degrees. Butter your baking sheet liberally.

In a medium-sized bowl stir together almond meal, salt, garlic powder or fresh garlic, and herbs.

In a small bowl beat eggs. Whisk in butter or coconut oil.

Pour wet ingredients into dry. Mix well with a fork. Knead a few times in the bowl until dough comes together well. Shape the dough into a circle.

Place the dough circle on the buttered cookie sheet and press the dough into the baking sheet, working from the center out. Keep working to spread the dough as thinly and evenly as possible. It will not be perfectly even so let go of that and then finish as best as you can.

Now use a sharp knife to cut the dough into 1 ½ inch squares. Next use a fork to pierce each cracker twice.

Note: if you wish for a thinner cracker put the dough ball between two sheets of parchment paper and roll it out with a rolling pin to desired thinness. Take the top layer of parchment paper off and, grabbing by the corners of the bottom parchment paper, lay the paper and crackers on the baking sheet to bake. Use the same method to cut but be careful not to cut through the paper, and pierce with the fork. Cooking time might vary within 5 minutes or so depending on your oven. Watch them closely; you want them brown, not burnt.

Bake at 350 degrees for 11–15 minutes or until golden brown around the edges. Place on a cooling rack. If you ended up with some thicker crackers towards the middle, remove the thinner, browner crackers and place the remaining thicker crackers back in the oven for an additional 5 minutes or until crisp and firm.

Basic Bone Broth...

Crockpot method...(for 6qt crockpot)
(You can use any kind of bones and below are the most common and easily found.)

> *Beef:* 1 pound of beef bones, any combo, and 1 beef liver

Chicken: 1 chicken carcass or whatever chicken bones you have, plus 3–4 chicken feet and 2–3 chicken livers

Fish: 1 medium fish carcass with bones, head, fins, guts if possible

Optional: roast bones if they are raw for 30 minutes (5–10 minutes for fish) or until browned and smelling irresistible, at 450 degrees before adding to crockpot for deeper flavor

2–4 large cloves garlic, in skin is fine (if sharing your bone broth with pets, use 1-2 cloves only)

2 tablespoons fresh rosemary, 1 heaping teaspoon dried

1 tablespoon apple cider vinegar

Sea or pink Himalayan salt (to taste) (if sharing with your pet add salt after cooked when reheating or using in recipe)

Filtered water to fill crockpot

Add all ingredients to a medium sized crockpot, approximately 6 quarts, cover with water to within 2 inches from rim and set for 10 hours on low (for fish set to 4 hours). After the first round for beef reset timer for another 8–10 hours on low, for chicken reset for another 4–6 hours on low. You can leave it on warm for a few hours if you are going to use it shortly. Otherwise turn it off, strain and pour clear broth into quart mason jars to cool and store in fridge. I strain it while it's hot so as to get the fat and gelatin in the broth. If you wish to freeze some, cool completely after strained, then transfer to a freezer container or stainless steel ice cube tray(s) and voila – you are all set.

Basic Fresh Raw Coconut Milk...

Serves: 4–6

2 young coconuts – this is important (You will want to make sure you select the right coconuts. The younger coconuts have

soft flesh on the inside. In the older ones, the flesh has hardened which you do not want.)
Dash of sea or pink Himalayan salt (optional)
1 teaspoon raw honey (helps preserve it is not using all right away)

Break open your coconuts. You can use a heavy cleaver to do so but my new favorite tool is the **Coco-jack** – love it!!
Pour the liquid into the blender – make sure that you have strained out any pieces of coconut shell or husk that may be in the liquid.
Scoop out the flesh with a spoon or Coco-jack scraper and add it to the blender.
Blend on high for several minutes until smooth and creamy.
Add a dash of salt and the honey if using.
Blend again for 10 seconds, then transfer your milk to a jar or container and store in the fridge! Lasts for up to 3 days.

If no fresh young coconuts are available to you try this...

Coconut Milk Using Unsweetened Shredded Coconut...
Serves: 4-6
> 4 cups of filtered water
> 1 ½ -2 cups of unsweetened shredded coconut

Heat the water, but don't boil it. You want it hot, but not scalding.
Add coconut to a high-speed blender, then add the hot water. (If it doesn't all fit, you can add the water in two batches.)
Blend on high for several minutes until thick and creamy.
Pour through a fine mesh strainer first to get most of the coconut out, and if there are still too many solids for you, squeeze it a second time through a towel or several thicknesses of cheesecloth to get the rest

of the pieces of coconut out. Personally, I don't usually strain it; I like my milks pulpy and skipping this step saves time and energy.
If you had to split the water, put all the coconut that you strained out back in the blender, add the remaining water, and repeat.
Drink immediately or store in the fridge. Should be used within 3-4 days after making for best flavor and texture. Since there are no preservatives or fillers, the "cream" of the coconut milk may separate on the top if stored in the fridge. Just shake or stir before using.

Note: if you do strain it then spread your coconut pulp out on a dehydrator tray or baking sheet and place in dehydrator or in your oven at 180 degrees to remove the rest of the moisture. Once all the moisture has been removed, you now have coconut flour which you can run through your food processor for a finer grind. Store in a cool, dry place in a glass container.

Einkorn Water Kefir Bread...

(Einkorn is nonhybridized heirloom wheat which is higher in nutrition, very low in gluten and more digestible and well tolerated than any other type of wheat. Fermenting it breaks it down even further and removes more gluten.) If you do eat wheat this is one of the kinds it should be and how you should do it:

> 3 ½ cups organic all-purpose Einkorn flour, sifted
> 1 ½ teaspoons sea salt or pink Himalayan
> ¾ cup warm, chlorine-free, filtered water
> ¾ cup plain water kefir (you can substitute kombucha)

In a large glass bowl combine flour, salt, water and water kefir (or kombucha). Stir well to blend ingredients. Dough should be a ball that holds together; you don't want it too loose or wet. This dough will rise so make sure there is enough room in the bowl for this.

Let sit at room temperature (preferably between 60-75 degrees Fahrenheit or 13.9-15.5 degrees Celsius) for 24–30 hours. No need to stir or mix during this time unless you happen to notice water sitting at the bottom of the bowl, at which point you should mix with a silicone spatula and refold back to a ball again.

After it has fermented for its allotted time, fold it one more time and turn on your oven to preheat to 350 degrees. Grease your baking pan liberally with coconut oil, ghee or butter.

Pour the dough into your well-oiled baking pan and smooth it out. Bake for 55 minutes or until the bread feels firm on top and bounces back when you press on it from the top and comes out clean when you poke it with a toothpick. It should also be browned nicely on top. Remove from the oven, then from the pan, and place it on a cooling rack. Let cool to room temperature, then store in the fridge or freeze for future use. Of course, you can always cut a slice off for yourself and slather it in butter to taste it after it has cooled slightly.

My Favorite Shopping Resources
Here are the links to some of my favorite resources for everything from recipes to products and so much more...

I actually order quite a few staple items from Amazon. And in case you can't find them locally, here are some of those items:

Dulse flakes

Maca powder

Yogurt starter

Matcha powder

Raw cacao powder

Unpasteurized miso (I prefer South River Miso but use this for those months they don't ship and I run out)

Wheat free tamari

Nama shoyu

Nutritional yeast

Raw Honey

Coconut sugar

Raw cane sugar

Organic maple syrup

Ghee

Grass-fed butter (This link is for multiple packs of Kerrygold; best deal on Amazon; share with friend or freeze). (If you live near a Trader Joe's or Whole Foods in the US, you will find a lower price there on Kerrygold butter.) (Any true grass-fed butter is fine too; look for local providers at your farmers market.)

Red palm oil (which I use for baking occasionally; this brand does not contribute to deforestation)

Duck fat

Grass-fed lard and tallow

Einkorn flour

Thrive Market is another resource for many of the items listed above and others at great deals. *

Olive oil you can trust to be real and not mixed with vegetable oils - Olea

This is my favorite and the BEST miso I have ever found and tried – South River Miso

The only coconut oil I recommend because of its quality and purity, oh and did I mention awesome taste?! – Skinny Coconut Oil*

A resource for sprouted nuts, seeds, nut butters and sprouted grains and flours – Blue Mountain Organics*

For water kefir grains, kombucha starter, yogurt starter and so much more – Cultures For Health.

Real foods, raw, fermented and so much more – Wise Choice Market*. Note: Wise Choice Market has cultured, fermented veggies, juices and bone broth too.

For the most wonderful teas (love their Chorus Dawn; blend of green rooibos, nettle and rose petals), essential oils, organic herbs and spices and more – Mountain Rose Herbs*.

For skincare, haircare and pets – Isvara Organics

The **ONLY** (seriously it's the only one I know of that will support your oral microbiome and it's fabulous!) toothpaste I recommend because it supports your oral microbiome – Revitin (available for sale fall 2015!)

Tool to open your coconuts – which I now love to do! – Coco-jack*

If opening coconuts is not for you, this is the only packaged coconut water that I recommend – Harmless Coconut Water use their locator to find where to buy it.

Line of water filter, shower filter, bath filter I use – New Wave Enviro – Water filter, shower filter, bath filter

*Affiliate Disclosure:

Because I wish to be completely transparent, these links marked with an asterisk I have an affiliate connection to. When you purchase something from these links you are supporting *I Live Vibrantly* to continue producing quality material for your education, such as this book.

I only link to products/sites I personally use and recommend to my clients. I believe whole-heartedly in all the items I have listed in this resources section whether affiliate or not.

My goal in sharing these resources, both product and information, is to support you to Live Vibrantly! with ease and discover new things.

Recipes, information and interesting reads:

My friend and colleague – Sarica

Food Renegade

Nourished Kitchen

Nourishing Days

Holistic Squid

Mommypotamus

Healthy Home Economist

Meet "Doc" Wheelwright: Master Herbalist, Biochemist, Eclectic Healer, Philosopher

Born 1917 in Utah, USA

Died 1990 in Utah, USA

Doc had a background in biochemistry and nutritional theory. He was a scientific, creative genius of his day and left the legacy of pioneering an herbal triad system that stimulates support for the targeted health issue while concurrently providing aid to the other connecting body systems.

Doc spent more than 50 years researching and travelled round the world, literally walking into primitive areas to discover and learn from some of the world's oldest and most beneficial herbal practices including Native American herbology combined with the herbal traditions of China, India, Tibet, Africa, Polynesia, Brazil and Europe. He called these healers the barefoot doctors and spent much time with them in his travels. He believed that plants held the solutions to humanity's greatest health concerns. These herbal traditions became his foundation for a new dimension in nutrition and herbal healing based on both biochemistry and bioenergy. He believed plants support human life and impart elemental vitality for our continued life processes.

His lifelong nutritional research culminated in his creating a diet plan called "The Lo-Stress, 5+5 Diet". I have taken those principles and applied them to where we find ourselves as humans today; working to thrive in an environment that works against us on many levels. The principles outlined here in the *Live Vibrantly* 10 step blueprint are based on his lifelong research and traditional ways of humankind.

Doc was far ahead of his time with what he presented; science is only now starting to catch up. And as you know it's amazing for "nutrition information" to still be valid after several years in our ever-changing world. Doc's research and teachings are for us today just as life supporting as they were back then. I will even go so far as to say even more vital as we deal with environmental pollution, chemicals, pesticides, depleted soil, electromagnetic fields, lack of clean water and so much more.

I did not have the honor of meeting Doc in person, unfortunately, but I was blessed to meet Dr. Jack Tips in 2001, who had worked side by side with Doc and learned from him directly. The part that resonated the most with me as I learned and studied Doc's teachings was that the bioenergy found in plants would support humans to thrive at a cellular level. Hence life = life. How alive your food is = how alive you are. This is Doc's legacy, and my service is to share it with you so you can flourish in your life as is your birthright.

Supplementation:

There was a time years ago when supplementation was not necessary, as we could get all the nutrients we needed from our planet and its provisions. That time is not now. Our soils are too depleted. The air, rain, and water are polluted. Chemicals and pesticides abound. We are surrounded by electromagnetic fields almost everywhere we go. I believe foundational supplementation is necessary in our day and age and that, coupled with the bioavailable nutrients from our foods, can support one to thrive and flourish.

I am referring to maintenance here and not therapy which is a whole separate category and depends on what the individual needs are. I recommend the following as part of your basic foundation:

100% herbal whole food cellular multivitamin/mineral complex
Vitamin D3 with K
Essential fatty acid complex
Dosage will depend on what brand and kind you are taking

I prefer to use and recommend Doc's legacy of herbal and nutritional formulas for this supplemental foundation. I've made it easy for you and put it all together in a package you can purchase here as a one-month supply in my online store.

What to look for in your supplements:
- 100% whole foods and herbs, preferably raw, not pharmaceutical lab manufactured components bound to fillers and yeasts
- Come from a transparent source you can trust

Supplements are just that; a supplement to the nutrients you get from your food. Quality really counts. Know your sources, do your research before you purchase.

Pharmaceutical lab manufactured supplements are manufactured chemicals. Your body has a hard time recognizing them and after taking these for a while stress can occur within the liver and kidneys. You are better off not supplementing at all if quality supplements are not in your budget. If this is the case, stick with high quality food and focus on superfoods in your food intake. If you have to choose one, make that choice spirulina. It's rich in vitamins and minerals.

Following are the top 10 risks you need to be aware of when self-supplementing, and why self-supplementation is not recommended. These risks vary from wasting money to severe drug interactions and nutrient depletion.

1. Self-supplementing can be just as dangerous as self-prescribing or self-diagnosing.
2. Health food store employees often don't have education or experience in clinical nutrition.
3. Labels can be deceiving and confusing.
4. There are more products out there with negligible doses than with appropriate doses; don't be fooled.
5. Not all supplements and vitamins are safe; some are absolutely contraindicated for certain people.
6. The media (news, TV shows, internet, etc...) are more interested in thrilling an audience than doing legitimate research.
7. Don't believe everything you hear; when in doubt ask a nutrition expert you trust.

8. Some supplements are targeted towards specific populations or conditions but when you look at the ingredients they're just repackaging a multivitamin or a single nutrient, calling it something else and charging way too much.

9. I would prefer a world where everyone got their nutrients through whole foods. As mentioned, this is not possible for most in this day and age, especially for those who have digestive issues, are deficient or don't eat enough whole foods. These people especially should be taking appropriate supplements.

10. If you're going to be spending hundreds or thousands of dollars on supplements each year, it would serve you well to know which ones are necessary and which are not.

- There are some great companies out there, such as the professional lines I use in my practice, that take into consideration the quality and source of their herbs and vitamins, proper dosage, common allergens and sensitivities, toxicity, and harmful fillers, among other important aspects. Those are the companies you wish to support, not the "in it for a buck" ones who are selling terribly made supplements. Because I do not use over-the-counter supplements, I'm not familiar with what's out there anymore. One that I can recommend, though, is Eclectic Institute for ethics, purity and source.

Here's to you Living Vibrantly!

60261615R00082

Made in the USA
Middletown, DE
28 December 2017